My Life My Canvas
My Way

JoEllen Koerner

Published by My Life My Canvas

Sioux Falls, South Dakota

www.mylifemycanvas.com

Acknowledgments

Grateful acknowledgments are made to the countless patients and families who shared their stories and lives with me in a moment of crisis or vulnerability. The courage and resourcefulness with which they faced adversity has been a constant sense of inspiration and hope in my life

Cover by Kristi Welch

Printed and bound by CreateSpace, an Amazon Company

ISBN: 1492700096
ISBN-13: 978-1492700098

DEDICATION

The creative spark of life, this instinctive motivation for growth towards self-realization, resides in the heart of humanity. Five decades of nursing practice in our richly diverse and complex society revealed that there are as many different paths towards authenticity as there are people—each life is unique. Yet this essence of being human unites us all. It is to this central core, which carries the continuity of our being, that this work is dedicated.

CONTENTS

PREFACE

<u>Who I am Depends on Me</u>

Patty Hendrickson

I am a human being.
I will fail, but I am not a failure.

There is good and bad in this world.
I will do bad things, but I am not bad.

There are right and wrong answers.
I will give wrong answers, but I am not wrong.

I am a collection if ideas, impressions and experiences.
I act upon this collection.

Every creature is a different collection.
We act differently. That is OK.

My failure may be your success.
My bad deed may be your good deed.

My wrong answer may be your right answer.
It's OK. We are different.

I am only responsible for one human being—me.
I know only one collection—my own.

Who I am depends on me.

INTRODUCTION

The alarm clock has gone off—ringing wildly in our ears! We grope for the off switch, stumble out of our sleepy state and take a good long look in the mirror. What do we see? A society at the crossroads—a turning point in human history. Which way we go will depend on how we define and understand ourselves and the possibilities that lay ahead. We have to start where we are, as we are, with our ordinary everyday selves, living each moment with conscious awareness, purposefully making small choices that lead to large outcomes. They create our masterpiece—our life!

The health of society is in a fragile state, as is the condition of the earth. Studies and outcomes point to unprecedented rates of obesity, chronic illness, and disability. Emotionally, the papers are filled with stories of depression, anger, violence and suicide. Socially, long-standing institutions and processes are faced with issues too large to solve in a simple and straightforward manner. And spiritually, for many, materialism is the god to be worshiped.

Lest we lose heart, we simply have to shift our gaze slightly—and we notice a beautiful and growing body of individuals, groups and systems, that have globally redefined who they are, what they are doing and where they are going. Within that collected group and their activities, a new world is being born.

The suffering of humanity is not new. Nor is the resolve of the human spirit to transcend and recreate the world. Having spent my entire career in nursing, I have had the privilege to witness the human spirit in times of great joy and sorrow. Supporting an individual or family, in all their courage and brokenness as they sort through the challenges of the day in response to a crisis, is a privilege of magnitude. It has been both instructive and inspiring.

What my many patients have taught me is this: *'What I see, know and understand, guides my life and actions. What I believe is possible is as far as I can go'.* I have seen two people with similar conditions end up with very different outcomes, though the opportunities were comparable for both. The human condition is a fragile and beautiful state: the universal life impulse is towards greater understanding of oneself and the world. Each situation, whether invited or imposed, holds a great lesson that can deepen our awareness and our capacity for a fuller life *if* we grasp the meaning in the event. But to do so we must be open and curious, flexible and adaptable, experimental in nature and able to recognize what is before us as well as within us. Fear, anger, scarcity, and low self-esteem, are all barriers to human unfolding. While these things are true for some—the one variable that stops us all is—a lack of conscious awareness.

How many of the beliefs and attitudes you hold today are your own? Think of all the rules and duties we carry around that come from others: early childhood culture; authority figures at home and work; community and government leaders; professional experts such as physicians and lawyers; and the always-present media shouting in our ears. It is very difficult to hear the still small inner voice of your own whispering wisdom, hard earned from a life time of experiences. How we reconnect with our own understanding, our own soul and spirit, is the main focus of this book. For only when you are connected to yourSelf do you create your own life story, instead of giving the job to someone else. Authenticity demands that you show up—for YOU!

Changes in science and technology are bombarding the world of health and wellness. It is easy to get lost in the multiple choices for managing diet, exercise, stress, etc. As our society gets increasingly diverse—in culture, beliefs, and practices—it gets harder to find 'the one right answer' or the 'one right way'. Nursing is a sacred privilege. Through many years of practice, it became evident that underlying our religious, social and political differences resides a pattern of similarities that are deeper than the social order of the day.

When physical, financial or relationship challenges come into our life, the fundamental longing of the heart, which fuels the human soul, is for truth, beauty and goodness in our life and the world. Pettiness falls away as we search for the basic meaning in life. This is our universal field of connection.

Early last year I was introduced to the work of Rudolf Steiner, and my understanding of life shifted. A framework for how to weave western, eastern, and middle-east beliefs and health practices into a coherent whole emerged. Suddenly a sense of comprehension and clarity filled my understanding. With this broader view of what it means to be human, I found room for all varieties of individuals; the unique traditions and expectations of patients, families and communities, and the spiritual beliefs they held. It also set the table for health care practitioners and lay caregivers alike, with various backgrounds and skills, to share their talents and contributions in an environment of respect and collaboration..

A new sense of connection and relationship enriched my enlarging awareness. A greater freedom of spirit filled me as I revisited the mental models I had been carrying about being human, about health, about life, about death. Old and worn out beliefs were exchanged for broader and more inclusive ones. Suddenly all the challenges, judgments and struggles regarding how to support diversity fell away as I understood things at this higher level of order. A peace that transcends understanding became mine. It is those models, and insights that enhance understanding I would like to share with you in this book.

Rudolf Steiner (1861-1925) was an exceptional science/philosopher. His unique genius was an ability to translate the ancient human striving to know ourselves into modern language and awareness. This dedicated servant of humanity combined spiritual research with the contemporary science of his age. Extensive in its practical implications for daily living, his work was based on history, physics, mathematics, biology, psychology, astronomy and spiritual principles. From this broad foundation his work is making a significant global impact on education (Waldorf Schools), agriculture (biodynamics) and medicine (anthroposophic medicine). A man with far-reaching capabilities, Rudolf Steiner was also an artist, a playwright and an architect. Above all, he was a world-transforming thinker, similar to other luminaries such as Aristotle and Thomas Aquinas. Through his research, observations, writings and lectures he created for us—*a path of knowing*.

Do you remember your years as a teenager when your parents, who had your best interests in mind of course, would ask; *Who do you think you are? Where have you been? What are you doing?* We would mumble some incoherent response because—in truth—we were not always sure how to answer those probing questions. This book is divided into three sections, each of them designed to explore one of those questions as they relate to your life and its quality. A model of the topic under consideration is presented to give a common framework for our consideration. A series of tools and processes help examine themes and concepts in the context of your life. Each chapter finishes with examples or stories that illustrate their application in daily life.

This book is simply a small introduction to a very large body of work that has emerged from the wisdom and inspiration of Rudolf Steiner, as well as some of the basic belief structures of various cultures. Each chapter can be read in 'stand-alone' fashion. Each section can be read without needing to explore the section which precedes or follows it. Pick a thought, a topic or a field of inquiry and start there— no need to read cover to cover.

An extensive recommended reading list is found at the back of the book so that you can continue down the 'path of knowing' on your own. I assure you that after taking this first step—you won't be able to stop. Without looking back you will press on towards your own destiny, connecting with your authentic self in all its beauty and fullness, making the human journey in general, and your biography in particular, an epic masterpiece!

Part I

My Life: Being Human
Who do you think you are?

We must want to be human as well as efficient, to be loving as well as informed; to be caring as well as knowledgeable; to be happy as well as respected. We choose and act, not in the light of what is good for me, but what is good for us. It brings growth to the entire human community.

Joan Chittister

CHAPTER 1

Being Human:
The 'Whole' of It!

The main thing in life is to not be afraid
of being human.
Aaron Carter

W HO ARE YOU?? A human life is a work of art
which each person creates uniquely. Each of us
has an 'idea' about what makes up a human being.
Some folks think of themselves as a body moving around the
world, guided by instincts, needs and desires. Others are
more focused on thoughts and opinions that guide their
choices and their life. Still others are on a 'quest'....a
pilgrimage seeking meaning and purpose in everything they
do. And who is right? Every single one of them! Complex
relationships exist between how we think, feel and act. When
we fully understand all the rich layers and textures of who we
are, balanced wholeness creates joy, peace and beauty in our
life and the world.

Every artist needs paints and brushes, the tools of their
creation. You come equipped with a physical body, an
emotional soul and a thought-full spirit. Your uniquely
inherited tendencies and abilities, personality, dreams and
goals are the substance of your being—*My Life*. The first
section of this book will explore what it means to be human,

to be healthy, and how your GPS sensory system guides your navigation in the world. A Model for Being Human addresses four basic characteristics that make you who you are (visible and unseen). Three coordinating life processes are always interacting and influencing your life at every moment; body, emotions and mind. All three must be considered together when making a choice or trying to understand.

Birth grants each of us a unique destiny with unlimited options for discovering and expressing it—***My Canvas***. The middle section of this book will explore the stages and patterns of your biography, and the meaning it holds for you. All human beings pass through universal stages of development in life that offer opportunities for growth and change physically, mentally, emotionally and spiritually. From impressions and experiences you evaluate and make choices each day as you create your own biography—your own 'I' history. A Model for Biographical Development examines the universal phases of life; how each seven-year period has its own point of view, its own purpose. To uncover the patterns in your biography, accepting and understanding them, is one of the most challenging issues of life and key to successful aging. When we can understand all parts of ourselves, we naturally understand others as well.

Every living thing is part of an even greater system that interacts in rhythms and cycles of life. From days of the week to seasons of the year, we are in constant exchange with others. The art of mindful awareness fosters right choices that help us establish and maintain inner and outer harmony and balance—***My Way***. The final section of this book will explore ways to construct your days to maximize a balanced life filled with quality and joy. From an aware and informed understanding we can make choices that improve our health and wellbeing, our mental and emotional development, moving us towards wisdom and peace in our old age.

A MODEL FOR BEING HUMAN

A model is a picture of different elements and their relationship to each other. It also demonstrates how they work together. The Model of Complete (Anthroposophic) Medicine is a universal holistic model being utilized around the world. Developed by Rudolph Steiner (see Introduction), it identifies fourfold human nature and how together these characteristics influence thinking, feeling and acting —it is a model of wholeness.

> *Humanity is made up of a material/physical body, a vital/energy body, an emotional/soul body, and a self-aware mind/ 'I' spirit. In health these four bodies must be seen and understood. In disease, disturbances must be observed and balance once more restored.*
>
> Rudolf Steiner

Fourfold Human Being:

The world is filled with multiple forms of life, human life being one of them. Because we are citizens of this earth we share many things with the rest of nature. We also possess something distinct from other life forms; we are the only species with a conscious self-aware mind. The Human Being is made up of four distinct and integrated 'bodies'. The different ways in which they interact gives rise to the uniqueness of the individual person. The four bodies include:

The Four Fold Human Being

Human Principle	Physical Body	Vital Life Body	Emotional Soul Body	Thinking 'I' Spirit Body
Characteristics	Form Space Weight Matter Size Shape	Breathing warming Nourishing Secreting Maintaining Growing Reproducing	Sensations Likes Dislikes Emotions Feelings Move on own	Autonomy Thinking Responsibility Moral Decisions Choices Meaning
Nature	Mineral	Plant	Animal	Human
Conscious Awareness	None	Sleeping Awareness	Dreaming Awareness	Waking Consciousness
Element	Solid (earth)	Fluid (water)	Flowing (air)	Warmth (fire)
Visibility	Visible	Invisible, effects seen on body over time	Invisible, effects seen in movement & actions	Invisible, effects seen in biography development

Adapted from Therakleine, 2003, p. 15

Your Material/Physical Body– shared with the mineral world: is made of the earth's elements of chemicals, minerals, water and clay. Everything mineral is subject to the force of gravity. In and of itself, it is inert or lifeless. Two qualities shared between physical material and the human body include:
- o It provides form and structure for standing upright as you navigate your life path
- o It experiences the physical world through your senses & interacts with the world through your actions

Your Vital Life/Energy Body—shared with the plant species: is a set of biological life processes fueled by energy from the sun (externally) and sun stored in food (internally). This rhythmic, pulsing force involved in the fluid of plants, animals and humans, fosters life, energy and vitality. Two qualities shared between the human being and plants include:
- o You experience a life cycle of birth to death
- o You have the ability to reproduce your own kind

Your Psychological/Emotional Body –shared with the animal species: is made up of a brain and central nervous system, bringing a certain level of responsive awareness. Impressions from the outer world are experienced, triggering a reaction leading to likes and dislikes. Two qualities shared between animal and humans:
- o You have the ability to move about on your own
- o You experience basic thoughts, drives, instincts and emotions

Your Self-Conscious Mind/ 'I' spirit—unique to the human being: is the conductor of your life and its experiences. This master mind of your existence guides, integrates and course-corrects your thoughts and actions across your life span. Two qualities that distinguish you from the rest of life on the earth include:
- o Individual self-awareness: your sense of 'I'
- o The ability to artistically choose and act, creating your life experiences & biography

Three Fold Human Processes:

Along with the characteristics of who we are as humans, there is an unseen coordinating effort amongst our 'bodies' that guides our life journey. The combination of Thinking (spirit), Feeling (soul) and Acting (body) provides our life with the impulse to move, develop and transform. The way these processes combine and interact creates the unique personality of each individual.

The Three Fold Human Process

Human Process	Physical Body	Emotional Soul	Thinking Spirit
Function	Acting	Feeling	Thinking
Focus	Hand	Heart	Head
Physiology	Generative: Metabolic System Limbs/Movement	Rhythmic: Respiratory Circulatory	Focused: Nervous System Senses
Impact	Highly developed physical senses focus attention on the outer world and link those impressions with clear thinking to foster right action	Open feelings give the necessary intuition to discern the truth of our thoughts and the goodness of our deeds	Clear thinking connected with reality creates an appropriate and meaningful choice leading to right outcomes
Maturity	Death by Completion	Peace of Soul	Wisdom of Life

Adapted from Camps, 2006, p.24

Creative tension must exist for growth and movement; status quo is death. When opposites (polarities) are influenced by a third force, new order is born. Your body and spirit are contrasting forces, with the soul bridging between them. Your Body is primarily made up of and focused on the 'Outer World'. Earthly matter, under the influence of the laws of the natural sciences, is filled with vital life processes that fuel metabolism and body movement. It is an organ of action, engaging the world to create experiences and opportunities for growth and contribution.

Spirit is primarily an agent of your 'Inner World' of values, thoughts, beliefs and intentions. Your mind's 'I'—insight, imagination and wisdom, coupled with your moral code or character, guides your *authentic self* in this realm. In this world your 'Higher Mind' (Spirit) envisions, creates, purposefully chooses and makes meaning. To access this world you need inwardness, quiet, and concentration.

The 'Middle Realm' is the home of your Soul; your world of emotionally influenced personality, intelligence and awareness. It builds bridges between the two opposing worlds; sometimes turned more towards earthly life (extroverted), and at other times turned inward (introverted). Just as our breathing and heart beats are in a permanent state of expansion or contraction, our feelings swing between positive and negative states.

At times the logic and reasoning of your 'Lower Mind' (ego-driven personality) is strongly influenced by instincts, feelings and desires—creating a swift emotional reaction— with outcomes that are not always positive. At other times, thoughts are less driven by feelings, and the daily intelligence of our *reliable self,* acts logically, drawing heavily on learned and patterned responses. Initially, strong emotions and desires dominate over thoughts and knowledge. One-sided thinking, separated from emotional warmth, can become cold and ruthless. One-sided acting, separated from clear thinking, can become chaotic or destructive. Only when our thoughts and actions mutually influence each other through balanced emotions do they become human.

As we mature, we begin to trust insights gained from our life experiences more than outer rules or unruly emotions. A shift in focus finds us increasingly trusting our intuition and growing inner awareness. We now come to experience our 'Higher Mind , the repository for the *Wisdom of Life—our life.* This *authentic self* can be cultivated by every person, regardless of rank, class or degree of learning,. It is developed as the body moves from youth, to maturity through aging. The youthful imaginative mind is accompanied by the lack of patience to wait, and the inability to see things in perspective, leading to hasty decisions. In later years this is replaced with wisdom, coming not from outer-directed activity, but from lessons learned from our varied life experiences. We develop the restraint of being able to 'wait and see' coupled with active *Peace of Soul*. The soul moves from being introverted or extroverted to a state of quiet. We put our emotions to rest, silence habitual thoughts and reactions, and have no lingering deep fears or desires. We have lived long enough to develop trust that the process of life will eventually resolve all issues; goodness reigns.

Each moment that we spend becoming aware of our 'negative inner talk'—derogatory, judgmental and critical opinions of others that are still in our mind—we get closer to truth. Filling our thoughts with understanding and respect for the world, uncluttered with projections or aversions, awakens forces that lie unused. We begin to see things around us that we could not see before; we had been seeing only part of the world through a judging and limiting lens. Now we can see our fellow human beings and all we experience in a more complete way, deepening our joy and appreciation for all of life.

A MODEL FOR HUMAN DEVELOPMENT

Life is designed in cycles and stages of development; we move from past to future in a constant process of transformation. Aging is a container for experiencing developmental change. While every person's path in life is unique, an individual work in progress, every single human being meets certain milestones throughout life which are universal in nature. Regardless of our background, critical outer and inner stages must be completed as we move through our life. How we meet them and travel through them paints the unique and magnificent masterpiece called 'My Life'. Our individual biography is the portrait which is personally and uniquely created by each one of us, highlighting the challenges and outcomes of that journey.

Development is different from change (things moving in a stream of time) or growth (an increase in number or size). It is '*blueprinted growth*' in which changes in structure occur at critical moments throughout the whole system. Human development is directed towards an end; the predetermined cycles of a human life and the maturing of the spirit. The cycles of birth, maturation and decline are programmed into all living organisms, including humans. In specific stages, the entire system (person) outgrows the capacity of their old self and must transform into something more or it will disintegrate. Good health, peace of mind and happiness are the fruits of stable development.

Universal Stages of Development:

A human life can be divided into four main categories (the fourth stage is possible if longevity is experienced):

Biological Development is the main characteristic of the first phase of human life. It is the stage of preparation. The primary task of this age (conception – 21) is to build our body and allow the organs to mature (Biological Curve). We do not contribute a great deal to our destiny at this time. Taking and receiving is a characteristic of this stage.

Emotional/Soul Development is the middle phase of life. It is the stage of expansion (21-42). Here the major task is self-education and self-development. Our personality, tightly tied to our body in phase 1, now 'comes of age' so we are able to determine and be responsible for the course of our life. Here we establish a family, a home, and a career. We develop social connections, taking our cues from other people. We experience a multitude of emotions; confrontation, love, enthusiasm, antagonism from others. We must learn to live with our feelings and bring our ego under control. Through all these existential battles our soul is refined and we achieve psychological (emotional curve) maturity. Generative and degenerative bodily forces are balanced at this point. We develop ourselves as 'individuals' in the world; we are now physically strong and emotionally stable—we are grown up. Giving and taking marks the struggles and joys of this stage.

Mind/Spirit Development is the third major stage of life in which the fruits of our life become visible. This is the stage of maturing (42-63). Our biological forces begin to gradually weaken; degenerative forces gain the upper hand. We move from a deep personal focus to setting objectives in the larger context of society. Our vital life energy shifts from supporting our physical body (menopause & aging) to strengthening our soul and spirit. The rules of hierarchy and dictates of others fall away as our authentic voice is heard more clearly if we choose to work on inner development. We become more morally and spiritually refined, less concerned about material things. If we do not do the inner work our body can become prey to the degenerative forces. The emphasis shifts to giving in this phase; the time of human fulfillment.

Integration & Completion is a final stage in life for those who live into advanced years. It is the stage of joy and peace (63++). While physical strength declines, a deep sense of understanding is felt. Young children experience joy because they do not yet know anything. Elders experience joy from a place of wisdom—they now know that struggles will eventually be resolved, and that what matters in the end is love. The beauty in simple things is seen and appreciated with wonder and gratitude; as when they were young. Having done the inner work of putting things and relationships in order to resolve the key issues in their life, a deep sense of peace pervades their final years. They end their life with 'death by completion'.

Human Development Curve

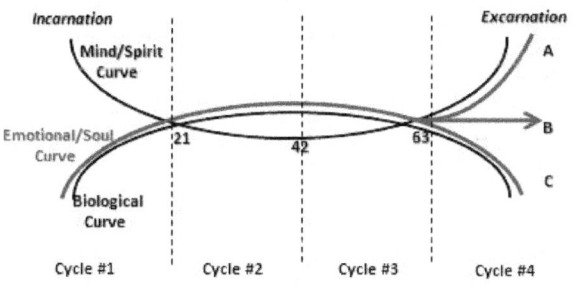

Adapted from G. Burkhard, p.20, 2011

Since human beings are not only physical, but also soul and spirit, there is great developmental potential in the second half of life. "Life begins at 40" has truth in it. The first half of life is fairly well defined by developmental laws and social norms. However, the activities and outcomes of the second half—designed to move us increasingly towards our authentic self—is our choice. We make a decision (consciously or unconsciously) for one of three outcomes: we may choose to pursue self-knowledge and development (A) try to maintain the energy and activities that were important for the first half of life (B) become cynical and disillusioned; the warmth goes out of our life (C).

A Living Example of 'Complete' Health & Wholeness:

Where would you go to find the best example of healing and wholeness? One such case can be found in Berlin on the grounds which served as Hitler's Headquarters during WW II. This space supports a beautiful healing garden and hospital which produces some of the best clinical outcomes and patient satisfaction scores in all of Europe. Visiting their Cancer Center, one is able to identify how a collaborative team of clinicians and therapists identify and treat the Four Fold Human. An extensive biographical review is also undertaken to explore the thoughts, feelings, actions and intentions that guide their life.

Much of the Western world views the *human being as two-fold*; a thinking mind and physical body that *can be cured*. A cancer patient visiting a state-of-the-art cancer center in the United States gets exceptional care. Chemotherapy, radiation, guided imagery and nutrition are administered to support the recovery process. Side effects from the treatment are managed with other pharmacological and supportive care practices.

An integrative hospital focused on *'complete healing'* hospital offers treatment to the *four-fold human being*. A cancer patient visiting one of these hospitals in Europe (also found in many other locations in the world, including select sites in USA) has a broader experience. Upon entering the hospital with a diagnosis of cancer, the Physical Body is treated with chemotherapy, as in conventional medicine. However, once the treatment has begun, the patient is taken out to a healing garden to address the Vital/Life Body. Here the gardener introduces the plant mistletoe, showing the qualities and properties of the plant and how they relate to the same aspects in a physical body. The assets of this plant strengthen basic cell health, potentiating the cell's inherent capacity for self-healing. The patient will receive both medications simultaneously; one destroys the cancer while the second enhances the self-healing capacity of the body, drastically minimizing side effects from the chemotherapy.

The patient is also given an organic diet and carefully selected nutritional supplements based on the unique state of the patient's health. Hydrotherapy and body massage also enhance the energy exchange within the body, strengthening and energizing the 7 biological life processes which manage the body's functioning (breathing, warming, nutrition, secretion, maintenance, growth and reproduction).

The patient then moves to the Art Room. The Emotional/Soul Body finds expression and comfort through various art forms (emotional language is sound and symbols). If the disease is 'hot', such as a psychosis, clay is given for sculpting. From the earth, clay is cool and grounding, a perfect medium for an ungrounded episode. If the disease is 'cool' such as cancer or depression, the patient is provided with warm yarns and paint colors to design a symbol or image depicting their emotional world. Working with such mediums expresses and releases pent up emotions and fears, further facilitating the self-healing capacity that resides within each of us—our body's internal wisdom.

After art class, the patient enters the Music Room. Vibrational energy from drums, bells, and various instruments help the natural rhythms of the body align and stabilize. Music sooths the soul and chaotic emotions. For those who are weak, a 'musical bed' provides a place for rest that wraps the body in an envelope of vibrating sound to strengthen the patient's own rhythmic pattern. This further aligns the patient's rhythms with those of nature coming from the sun and the center of the earth. All is potentiating the cells function and repair.

A final therapy for the day finds the patient in the Biography Room. The individuality or 'I' of the person holds the unifying thread woven throughout their whole life. However, biographical development takes place in rhythms of seven year periods. With the help of psychologists or spiritual counselors (depending on the belief system of the patient), the individual completes a life review that looks at significant events, choices and decisions within the 'developmental tasks' of the period in which it was experienced. Deeper insights and understanding about their personal patterns, passions and gifts help create a sense of authorship, authenticity and destiny in their life. Forgiveness and appreciation for self and other is enhanced; this facilitates healing.

A cancer patient comes to this experience with an illness, and leaves with a deeper sense of self-awareness. They have learned how to; care for their body, select energy-giving foods, have a deeper appreciation for nature, express and manage their emotions in an art form of their choosing. They also shed some of the betrayals, disappointments, and regrets they had carried, replacing them a sense of forgiveness and a deeper understanding about life and their place in it. This patient *may be healed on all levels of being.*

This example of caring for a cancer patient in a 'complete manner' is the blueprint for healthy living. While proper exercise, hygiene and nutrition are essential for health, equally important is the care and cultivation of your 'other bodies'. The remaining chapters of this book are dedicated to that end.

CHAPTER 2

Using Your Senses:
Making Connections

Common Sense is that which judges the
things given to it by the other senses.
Leonardo da Vinci

As a human being, you are a system in your own right.
However, you are only one living system nested in
with many others—each dependent on the rest for its
basic survival, relationship and meaning. All contact with the
outer world occurs through your senses. Classic science has
identified six ways in which you sense the outer world with
your physical and vital biological body; hearing, sight, touch,
taste, smell and balance.

Anthroposophic science compliments natural science with
another point of view, identifying and enlarging our
understanding of who we are with an additional set of 'senses'
that connect to our inner world. Rather than supporting a
physical function, these senses serve the human experience
itself such as a sense of our life vitality or awareness of our
own movement. As we develop more sensitive 'I' awareness,
these senses lead us towards maturing our emotional and
spiritual qualities. We then move into a right relationship
with others as we become present in ways that enhance the
relationship—and our biography.

A MODEL OF HUMAN SENSES

In the first half of life our senses serve to connect us to the outer world to gain experiences. At mid-life our orientation to the world and ourselves shifts inward. These same senses then take on the more subtle capacity of connecting us in a broader and more comprehensive way to the larger world (both inner and outer) so that greater sensitivity and wisdom is experienced. The twelve senses can be classified into three distinct groups.

#1- *Bodily Senses* – establish a relationship with your own body.

These four senses give insight and orientation to your body and its functioning. You can sense how well you are doing physically in the following ways; sense of touch, sense of life-energy, sense of your own movement and sense of balance. Every morning you 'check in' with your body to determine how much energy and vitality you have for the day. You may feel stiff and sore or flexible and fluid. The world spins out of control in dizzy fashion or you are centered like a rock. We continue to check in frequently during the day, mostly unconsciously, to determine 'how we are feeling'. This information helps us set boundaries and make choices to move forward or modify our original plans.

Sense of touch- functions via the skin. We experience touch by sensing pressure and resistance. Here we meet the border between ourselves and the world. We sense the relationship between our body and everything external to it. In the second half of life the ability to discern what is ours and what belongs to others requires the spiritual qualities of discernment and respect.

Sense of life- tells us whether our body is functioning harmoniously or not. When problems arise we may notice a headache, upset stomach, pain, sickness, or cramps in our body. Spiritually, through the experience of our own pain we come to understand the pain of others. This allows us to develop the capacity to be present to others, giving excellent service, comfort and support to others while also cultivating compassion.

Sense of movement- gives us a sense of direction in relation to the environment. We can change the position of different parts of our body without having to look whether our legs are crossed or our head is turned to the side. Just as we can move our body towards a desired path, with enhanced awareness we can focus our thoughts and actions to reach our life aims.

Sense of balance- helps us find our center when there is tension between the environment and ourselves. Only when we are in equilibrium, free of physical obstacles or emotional blocks such as fear or ego, can we experience our true center. By exercising balance, we can establish harmony between ourselves and the world.

The sense of touch separates you from the world; you are a bounded individual. The senses of life and self-movement give you information on how to physically navigate the world. And then, the sense of balance leads you to a right relationship with the world.

#2- *Social Senses* – establish relationships with your outer surroundings.

More than simply moving your body through life, these senses serve as a way for your emotional soul to express itself through your life relationships. When we connect with something in the material world, something also responds emotionally in our soul. What begins with a physical experience is enriched when we bring in emotions of the personality.

Sense of smell- Smells are always the result of a substance in the process of disintegration. It is a basis for personal hygiene. Scent compels us to make a judgment; both physical and moral. A sense of pleasant or unpleasant may increase or stop any further exploration. As we mature, we begin to suspend habitual judgment or rise above prejudice. This opens the door for discovering a real interest in things previously rejected, or a deeper understanding regarding the 'how' and 'what' of the unfamiliar. Often the most interesting and rewarding people and experiences appear 'different' from our old habits and patterns of thought.

Sense of taste- is an intimate matter—a two-way exchange. Taste gives us a qualitative direct experience with a substance (sweet, sour, bitter, or salty). We decide which elements go together (like wine and cheese pairing). We chew it over, make a conscious effort to spit out or swallow the contents so that they become something new in our body (physical growth or a new idea). When we taste something it has a lasting effect on us; it is something we become.

Sense of vision- extends us out into the world. Sight moves from darkness into light. All-embracing, vision encompasses other senses; it helps maintain balance, influences taste and emotions, and body-awareness. Through our eyes the world opens to us. Sight captures everything in one glance; we can see the whole. From a beautiful sunset we can experience a sudden sweeping emotion of joy or sorrow, wonder or worry, delight and appreciation. The soul is intimately connected to the attentive eye.

Sense of warmth- Temperature is the first human experience after birth, arising from a flow experience between environment and bare body. We register a sense of temperature every time something happens between us and the world. Cold has a chilling effect and makes things contract, excluding other things in the environment. Warmth, on the other hand, has an enthusing and engaging impact, inviting one in. Later in life the soul develops the capacity to intuitively sense into the deeper nature and warmth of a thing. This monitoring opens us to selective interests and expands us by what comes back. This is the source of true navigation of our destiny.

These four social senses are used to engage in creative exchange between our self and the surrounding world. They relate information about the environment that triggers certain feelings. Initially the exchange rests in our personal experience, while later in life we consider more deeply the experience of others as well. As we reflect on an exchange and make the choice to go forward or move away, we soul-fully create our reality—the biography of our life.

3- *Spiritual Senses* –The mindful human spirit is of higher order than the emotional soul:

Your soul is in a continuous dance with the world, reacting to it and doing what is needed. It builds bridges between your spirit and the outer world. Your spirit is your highest self. Here you are free of ego and external instincts, connected directly to universal understanding and the creativity and wisdom you have acquired from all your life experiences.

Sense of hearing- involves more than just receiving sound. Hearing plays the most crucial role in human communication and connection; it is a highly social endeavor. We hear what other people and external things are saying and bringing to us rather than merely a sound picked up by our physical body. To understand and be understood, we share a part of ourselves with others through communication. Pure sound, like clean air, deals with quality. It is necessary to quiet ones perceptions and prejudices if clear, rather than selective hearing is to occur. Being open and empty assures accuracy in communication.

Sense of language- Language communicates a message beyond what is heard. To understand the spoken word we are concerned with feelings as well as thoughts. We must disregard our own emotions and experiences so we can truly sense the essence of another's voice. When we listen intently to the spoken words of another; their speech, feelings, emotions and body gestures flow in various ways that move us emotionally. In this way we can come to identify the color, mood and feelings of the person speaking. We understand 'their language', whether we understand the words or not.

Sense of thought- focuses on the pattern of organized thinking. We all have a series of beliefs and assumptions that were obtained throughout our life. While speech has to do with the spoken word, listening carefully for the pattern of thought in what is being expressed helps us uncover the beliefs and expectations that lie behind the words. We can follow what is being said and comprehend its meaning to the person speaking. When we understand each other at this level, a true spirit of community and belonging occurs.

The sense of authenticity— 'I' of another- the most difficult aspect of life is finding the authenticity within ourselves and others. We can become aware of our self and the other, each as individuals in their own right. Once we learn where we stand ourselves, we are ready to engage with others, sensing the 'meaning' of what is being said for each person. It is here that you make a decision to follow their lead or stay with your own.

12 Senses By Category & Experience

GROUP	SENSE	EXPERIENCE
PHYSICAL BODY—Physical Senses (relating to own body)	Touch	Determine one's own boundaries
	Life Sense	Vitality, growth & decay of own body
	Self	Handling own body
	Movement	Gravitational orientation
	Balance	
EMOTION/SOUL—Social Senses (relating to outer surroundings)	Smell	Action/Will: Morality—good-bad
	Taste	Feeling: Quality—healthy-unhealthy
	Vision	Thinking: Choosing—yes-no
	Temperature	Emotion: Warmth—attention-interest
"I"/SPIRIT—Spiritual Senses (relating to invisible uniqueness contained within things/people)	Hearing	Personal meaning behind communication
	Language	Cultural meaning within communication
	Thought	Pattern of organized thinking Authentic
	Unique "I"	individuality of both parties

Adapted from Soesman, 2006, p. 1-95

The final four senses are underdeveloped in the current human experience. Rather than supporting a physical or emotional function, they serve the human experience itself. Using these senses you start to understand the 'inner world' of others as well as your own. You discover what is common and shared between all beings and then connect with the essential nature of everyone and everything in the universe in a sense of oneness

We bring various levels of 'awareness' to every experience we have, from connecting with a simple object such as a table, to the complex interactions that occurs within a group or team. The more 'senses' we utilize, the more 'complete' the encounter will be.

Examining A Table

- **Physical Level**—I can walk up to the table and explore its physical characteristics; size, shape, height.

- **Emotional/Soul Level**—I can see and 'appreciate' the beauty of the wood, the craftsmanship that built the table.

- **Individual/Spirit Level**—I can 'connect' with the table and in relationship will discover the unique characteristics of the table. Leaning on it, I find that one leg is too short, the table is not trustworthy.

Through the compelling work of Dr Rudolf Steiner, we begin to understand the senses as the foundation for a life well-lived. By bringing all of our senses to an experience consciously rather than through routine habit or the filter of borrowed beliefs, we begin to experience our life, and the entire world, in a deeper and more significant way. If humanity is to fully develop, individual and collectively, we need the freedom and courage to explore and cultivate all twelve senses. From this broader way of engaging with the world we will develop a civilization that fosters truth, beauty and greater good for all.

A MODEL FOR SENSE-ENABLED DECISIONS

As human beings we are citizens of three worlds. Physically we belong to and perceive our own body. Only we can tell how our body and vital life processes feel. Social senses, which are more emotional in nature, help us to relate to the outer world surrounding us. Independent of what our body feels physically, emotional activities are triggered by real or perceived events in the privacy of our own thoughts and attitudes. Spiritual senses guide us to into an authentic relationship with ourselves and others. Through the higher mind of our spirit we step outside ourselves and let things reveal to us what is significant for them, rather than us deciding what is important or what things mean for them.

Our various senses guide different aspects of a decision. The issue being decided is followed by the appropriate 'sense' and set of questions that helps us discern the answer. Ponder the following questions when making a 'sensible' decision.

#1- Bodily Senses—connection to self:

Setting Boundaries: Sense of Touch- it makes a difference whether I am touching something (intimacy) or something is touching me (boundaries). <u>Questions:</u> Who am I; where do I stop and the next thing begin? What is the nature of what I am touching; size, shape, texture, desirability etc.? What do I want to connect with—how closely? Answers help us with boundary setting.

Commitment Decisions: Life Sense – a surveillance system for our survival. <u>Questions:</u> How am I doing? How am I feeling? How far can I push myself? How much further can I/do I want to go? Answers help us with endurance and tenacity decisions.

Action Decisions: Self Movement Sense – we have a say in the direction that we are going. <u>Questions:</u> What am I doing? Where am I going? Why am I going there? What do I want to accomplish? Answers help identify the plan behind the action.

Authenticity: Sense of Balance – a mechanism to tell us how we stand in the world. <u>Questions:</u> How do I stand? What is my point of view? Where is the middle ground in this issue?

How do I keep centered? Answers foster authenticity and integrity in our actions.

#2- Social Senses—connection to world:

Significance: *Smell-* there is a strong interaction between smell and basic life drives. Questions: What does this smell like? What created this odor? What is its quality? How strong is the attraction/repulsion? Answers help us discern the good from the bad, the significant from the insignificant.

Value Decisions: *Taste-* is a determinant of quality. Questions: How much do I need or want this? Do I like it? Is it in my taste? What is it worth to achieve this outcome? How will this impact me and others over time? Answers help us share our life in good taste with the world, fulfilling our destiny.

Goal Decisions: *Vision-* allows us to reach out in an expression of curiosity. Questions: What am I looking for? What do I see? What will a move in this direction accomplish? Answers allow us to more clearly see before us suffering and beauty in all things, including ourselves, fostering self-compassion and compassion for others.

Interest: *Warmth-* arises from the experience of flow. Questions: What is the temperature of my feelings towards this (cold is chilling while warm is stimulating)? How much curiosity do I have about this? What about this warms my heart and interest? Answers show us the level of attention and interest, the affinity we have for the issue at hand.

#3- Spiritual Senses—connection to Universal Wisdom:

Clarity: *Hearing-* true hearing comes from the space of silence, disconnecting us from our own instincts. Questions: Who do I listen to? How do I interpret what I hear? How do I suspend my patterned thoughts and assumptions so I do not contaminate the message being received? Answers help us clearly 'hear' the message given by the other, rather than our interpretation of what their words mean. A deeper understanding and more appropriate and targeted response is achieved.

Message: _Language-_ emerges from a long cultural tradition and cannot be created by one person. <u>Questions:</u> What word patterns are used in the communication? What cultural messages are encoded in the language being used? What is the expression of the messenger? What is their body language conveying? Answers help us follow body gestures rather than just the words themselves, which identifies the color, mood and emotion of the person or group speaking.

Understanding: _Thought-_ our thoughts reflect our understanding of how things work. <u>Questions:</u> What is the meaning behind this for each of us? What assumptions and perceptions guide my thinking, and the thinking of the other? What beliefs have we each acquired from our lived experiences and how will that impact things going forward? Where do our thoughts align in agreement and where is there a gap in connecting? Answers help us understand and comprehend a 'picture' of what is being conveyed. This fosters deeper cultural awareness in a complex and diverse world.

Original Though: _The 'I' Identity of Another-_ We either speak with the authority and authorship of our own life, or we live in borrowed thoughts and ideas. <u>Questions:</u> Who is behind the thought I am expressing—the spoken/written word of the other? Whose ideas does this person represent? What are the assumptions that underlie them? Answers to these questions foster truth, influencing whether we should allow ourselves to be swayed by them or stay on our own path.

A Living Example of Making a Sense-able Decision:

Making a decision that honors every aspect of your being will engage you with opportunities that foster growth and insight—even if it is challenging. Shifting the goal from a narrow definition of success and getting it right to self – discovery changes the game plan. This story comes from a middle-aged river canoe guide exploring his beliefs and expectations while trying to learn how to white-water kayak.

"Any life designed to suck its very marrow out of you is going to encounter a certain amount of failure, disappointment. I'm trying to learn whitewater kayaking right now and it isn't going well. Others can do it. Fellow students, people like me who are just beginning, seem to have mastered the basics quickly. I've done a lot more paddling than them, albeit in a canoe, but I should be able to do this. Instead, I constantly find myself upside down in my kayak, headed downstream. I grab the release on my spray skirt and eject into the river. (If this was the air force, I'd be well on my way to cleaning them out of jets.) Rescue ropes are flung through the air. Other kayakers race to grab my boat and paddle before they disappear over the horizon. I drag my tired, wet self up on the shore. I get back in my kayak, wait my turn in line, try to exit the eddy once more, and once again flip. Three times so far. No one else flips. I think I know what I'm doing wrong but my body doesn't follow my mind's instructions.

Afterwards, lying in bed at night, tired, discouraged, I think about quitting, but I can't. I keep at this because it is a new way to experience wild water, and wild water is important in my life. If I give up, my life will lack a richness that it would otherwise have. And my opinion of myself will be just ever so slightly diminished.

And the people rescuing me are wonderful human beings. They are kindhearted people, deep people; people of real character. They love to paddle wild rivers. When I learn how to do this, I'll be welcome among them. And in the meantime, as long as I keep trying, put my heart in this, they offer kind words of encouragement. So even now I feel welcome among them. If I can't show them technique, I can still show them heart.

Others may learn in a few hours what may take me days or weeks or months, but eventually I'll learn how to do this. And when I do, on the other side of this discouragement and disappointment, will be a deeper, richer life. A closer connection to the spiritual source; to the life source that is wild water."

"Fail at something important to you
Fail at something you should be good at
Fail at something others find easy.
But if it is important to you
Important to a deep experience of life
Just keep going back for more.
Keep trying.
Put your heart in it.
Live deep. Suck all the marrow out.
Someday it will be too late to keep trying.
In the meantime, a bigger life awaits."

-Rod Mcguiver

CHAPTER 3

Navigating the World:
Personal Presence

If you wish to travel far and fast,
travel light. Take off all of your
envies, jealousies, unforgiving
selfishness and fears."
Cesare Pavese

You are a are a force: a powerful bundle of energy that takes up a unique space in the universe! You alone occupy the place on which you stand. There is no other like you. You have a presence that makes an impact on everyone and everything you come into connection with as you travel across your lifespan. What sort of an influence do you leave behind?

Life is filled with two separate but connected human functions; doing and being. Often we are busy doing things with and for our self and others as life is filled with daily activities at work, at home and out in the world. Our actions show others visibly what we are thinking. At other times we are simply present, being with others or a situation as a silent witness or support in the moment, saying or doing nothing at all; we are just 'hanging out'. In that space of being we radiate our frame of mind, our intentions; our inner essence.

Your presence is a blend of both doing and being; the degree to which you show up to life in all its varied forms.

A MODEL FOR BEING PRESENT

Those who have mastered the art of living weave both doing and being into every encounter—it is their way of being present in the world. In any situation, the more mindful we are of the other (human or nature) and their unique needs and expectations, the more presence we bring to the moment. When we choose to 'show up', our actions are accompanied by an awareness of not just a physical body, but the emotional soul and unique spirit of the other. Connections are stronger, sharing is more honest, understanding is deeper and both become more authentic in the exchange. This is the foundation for good relationships or great customer service. Practicing presence creates a vibrant, connected and meaning-full life.

Connecting With Your Environment

An important aspect of life is the environment in which you live. Your surroundings have a 'spirit' or feeling of their own. Sometimes we feel 'right at home' and other times we feel more like a fish out of water. Basically our environment is comprised of three major elements:

- o *Natural surroundings*: includes things from the earth and its climate all the way to your private room and its furnishings.
- o *Social environment*: includes things from the significant relationships in your life such as loved ones, relatives and friends to the broadest aspects of a global society.
- o *Spiritual environment*: includes things from personal values, beliefs and expectations to elements from your culture; art, philosophy, ethics and religion.

Each of these environments continuously influences your life experiences and further development.

The physical body & its environment: The material body takes elements from the earth to construct a physical body we can see, bump into, touch and take hold of. It also takes materials from the environment in the form of nutrition. A physician may measure the level of iron in your blood, or may evaluate the weight of the human body.

The material body obeys the laws of the physical world. It is subject to the laws of gravity and occupies a unique space where no other matter can be. Yet the body is also separate from the physical world and not subject entirely to its laws. It does not dissolve in rain or freeze in frost. During life your physical body maintains a distinct and separate existence on, but apart, from earth. Only with death does it stop being a 'body' and become one with the mineral world once again. The physical body you identify as yourself throughout life, is actually 'on loan' from the earth itself.

The vital body & its environment:: Life forces express themselves biologically in the rhythmic fluid portion of the body. It is not the fluid itself, but the energy generated by the sun that causes vital biological processes to function. Delicate chemical processes continuously bring about changing conditions in physical matter; flowing, pulsing, and streaming with dynamic forces that permeate your body with life. Every living thing on earth experiences the continuous flow of this vital life energy.

The vital life processes link all people with each other and all things living. When one person goes to work with a cold, eventually the whole office has a cough. What happens on a small scale also has significance for the whole earth. Dramatic shifts on natural life patterns such as deforestation and river diversions cause a breakdown of the ecological balance. Prosperity and excess for some fosters hunger and deprivation elsewhere.

A moral imperative for all of humanity is to care, not only for their own physical body and personal health, but for the health of the whole earth. Like the material body, the energy body is 'on loan' from the vital life forces running through the earth. Upon death we give up our life force and it returns to the general vital force of the earth's atmosphere.

The soul body & its environment: Each of us has an inner world comprised of emotions and instinctive drives. Our soul is the home of feelings and thoughts, influenced strongly by our twelve senses within, and the energy pulsing from the external world—including planetary bodies. Studies show that there is a dramatic increase in hospital deliveries, a spike of activity in mental institutions and police stations, when the moon is full. Our emotions are strongly influenced by our unique 'biorhythms' as well as our response to 'natural rhythms'.

A series of pulsing energy systems interact with each other. Energy fields from the sky keep our atmosphere steady. Magnetic fields from the sun regulate life rhythms of all living things. Fields radiating from the earth's core support our own vital life force. Fields generated by moving water or other natural forces support our own emotional fields. Sounds, artificial lights and other human fields (i.e., love, anger or hate coming from individuals or society at large) do everything from stimulating our DNA or endorphins to prevent depression, to causing us to experience insomnia and stress. Energetically, the vibrations of what you think, say and do impact every other thing in the universe.

Each living being is encapsulated in their own bioenergy field. Extending as far as your outstretched arms, your unique energy pattern radiates from you to touch everything in your personal environment. This bounded energy field serves several useful functions: a) protection to shield you from negative energy; b) filtering to let good energy in; and c) communication by transmitting subtle messages into the world to influence the things around you. You can increase your vitality, in real time, through the practice of yoga or tai chi, meditation, massage, homeopathy or acupuncture, to name a few energy practices available today.

It is the nature of human souls to form communities that can be based on shared interests or wider family relationships. Some Native traditions believe that prior to birth we plan for our next life's destiny. We agree to work in groups of 20-30 souls who will show up strategically at a specific point in our life to play a role that will deepen our understanding and ability to love. Sometimes the one who loves us most plays the most difficult role in our current life drama, which is why one does not hate their adversary—this may be their one true love.

During our life, as our 'spiritual family members' appear, there is a quickening, an instant sense of recognition that this person has a significant role to play in our life. And, as we complete the contract agreed upon prior to birth, the person will give us back the piece of our soul they have been safeguarding for this experience. If we recognize each family member and complete the work assigned, we receive back all of the pieces of our soul as we follow our path of destiny— and, for them, that is the meaning of spiritual wholeness.

The 'I' body & its environment: On earth, as independent personalities, we have an intelligence that makes our own choices, decisions and creations. The 'I' is the element that carries personal responsibility for those activities. It holds our spirit, our higher self which contains the intuition and wisdom gained throughout this lifetime. Indigenous and Eastern traditions believe in reincarnation; repeated earth lives. The 'I', or individual core of the human being comes to earth in order to have experiences and learn from them. With death, life has not finished, instead, a new form of existence begins in which the 'I' processes and evaluates the experiences of the life just completed, and integrates them fully, to be used in the next incarnation.

Viewed from this perspective, life is regarded as a day school, with other days/lifetimes to follow. The aim of these repeated earth lives is to perfect ourselves until we reach the next stage of development. Between lives we plan for that next lesson, making a series of selections to 'set the stage' for our further learning. We choose a geographic location to learn a 'meta-lesson' from the underlying culture, (i.e., democracy in America, wisdom in China etc.) We select a date of birth, giving us a sign of the zodiac to teach specific lessons in personality. Our experience with our parents will teach spiritual lessons as we inherit their strengths and weaknesses to compliment or highlight our own. And, finally, we select our 'spiritual family' (referenced above) to co-create significant experiences and relationships for our destiny in the upcoming lifetime.

From this point of view 'misfortune', 'illness, or 'bad luck' are not viewed as mere accidents. They are seen as important life experiences, a part of destiny designed to gain new capabilities, insights and recognitions. Significant events are the consequences of a long chain of past causes, as well as preparation to acquire new capacities for this, or later incarnations. From this perspective, the human being on earth is not the product of chance. Every physical lifetime is the result of a long history of development with all its problems and errors, but equally with all the gifts and opportunities. This world view requires a culture that honors the ability to make mistakes. Rather than a blaming culture. In a learning culture, individual, group, and societal mistakes are embraced as learning opportunities which lead to further development.

The 'I' differs greatly from the other parts of being human. Unlike the other bodies, individuality is not on loan; it is central to each human being—it's essence. Each spirit is a world of its own. It is one of the goals of all humanity to become aware of this inner authentic individuality and make it ever more a part of our daily experience. When we include this wakeful state in our daily presence, we are able to create new realities for ourselves and the world. This is the force behind the continuing development of humanity.

UNDERSTANDING YOUR TEMPERAMENT

Temperament is the manner of thinking, behaving and reacting characteristic of a specific person, revealed in their reaction to things in life. It includes mental capacity, physical characteristics, moral attitudes and the emotional way that we behave, especially towards other people. This combination of physical, mental and emotional traits is the natural predisposition we are born with; our natural way of thinking and behaving rather than something we learn. While our temperament has a genetic and biological basis, environmental factors and maturation modify our personality and expression of temperament over time.

Differences in Temperament:

Differences in temperament characteristics such as introversion or extroversion, thinking or feeling, slow and methodical rhythm vs. highly active and quick to respond, greatly influence and affect interactions and relationships. These striking variances in behavioral styles between individuals are important factors in family and work life relationships. Understanding temperament in general, and your own in particular, can help reframe your interpretation of the behavior of others, and your relationship with them. Mindfully making small and reasonable accommodations for individual differences, and utilizing your unique characteristics for the enhancement of group/team processes, creates harmony and high performance of everyone involved.

Temperament is determined through specific behavioral profiles. Many classification schemes for identifying it have been developed: Meyers-Briggs, DISC, Keirsey Temperament Sorter, etc. It is a helpful exercise to take one of these profiles to gain insight into your own temperament and how it interacts in relationships. Once we gain insight into our own behavior, we have a deeper understanding of the human condition—making us more tolerant and respectful of the nature and attributes of everyone we encounter on our life journey.

<u>Making Mindful Connections:</u>

Mindfulness is at the root of Buddhism, Taoism and many Native-American traditions.   It is an active and open state of attention. Being present in the moment, we live our life awake to the experience we are having. Life unfolds in the present moment but it is often missed as we live in a world that contributes to mental fragmentation, distraction, and stress. At work we fantasize about vacation and while on vacation we worry about the pile gathering on our desk. Memories of the past or concerns about the future constantly intrude on our thoughts in the present moment. Navigating life in mindless distraction is equivalent to texting while driving—we are simply not present.

To get better control of our mind and our life, finding a deeper sense of balance requires stepping out of the chaos to pause in the stillness of our inner world. We become mindful as we connect with our 'I' spirit—the observer within. Introspection involves the observation of our own emotional and mental processes. We become aware that we are not our thoughts as we witness them from this perspective. Through a reflective looking inward, we can observer ourselves and the moment with non-judgment; neither grasping nor pushing things away. We let things be as they are. Instead of letting life go by without living it, we become awake and aware of each experience just as it is—adding nothing nor taking anything away from it. It is what it is.

Cultivating a nonjudgmental awareness in mindful presence has many benefits. It reduces stress, boosts immunity, reduces chronic pain, lowers BP, and helps us cope with complexity. Mindful people establish better relationships, are happier, more exuberant, empathic and secure. Higher self-esteem fosters more acceptance of our own and others weaknesses. It reduces the impulsivity and reactivity that underlies depression, binge eating and attention problems. From this centered position we can hear negative feedback without feeling threatened. We fight less, becoming more accommodating and less defensive. We become a positive and life-enhancing presence in the world.

BALANCING YOUR RHYTHMS IN TIME

Human time is configured in many ways, made rhythmic by intervals and pauses at all levels of the Universe. Rhythm is vitality. Heart beat and respiration move in and out in consistent recurring fashion moment by moment. Sleeping and waking moves us from exhaustion to vibrant energy every day. What we experience as freshness and enthusiasm in the morning corresponds to the season of spring. The dark of night and a quieter introspective mood corresponds to mid-winter. Aligning our ordinary needs and tendencies to those of the natural world enhances coherence. When we notice and work with the rhythms of life—in the moment— we experience maximum vitality.

Rhythms, cycles and transitions are physical, emotional and spiritual in nature. Some follow 24 hour cycles, while others occur in phases across the lifespan. Found in all living things, they are determined by genetics, the environment and universal forces. When we become aware of, and in alignment with them, we are in congruence—we are in sync.

Rhythms

Unlike your physical body, which is solid and stationary, your vital life force and emotional soul are more like water; fluid and ever changing in a constant flow of movement. The soul swings back and forth between two extremes—your inner and outer worlds. We find stimulation and experience in the outer world and then return home, entirely centered within our self. The more you are able to withdraw into your own thoughts with a good book, a thoughtful quote, or a quiet moment of meditation—even for just a few minutes a day—the more you will be prepared to engage with others or nature as you move back out into the world.

Patterns of Sleep: All daily activities—movement, work and play, as well as ideas, thoughts and feelings—require energy. During the day we use a significant part of our vital life force for managing body functions. Other great uses of this precious energy are our sensory activities and thinking. By the end of the day the physical body is depleted; it suffers from exhaustion. We feel used up, tired and physically drained while our head feels 'stuffed up' with ideas and experiences of the day.

One of the most common patterns in the human experience is the sleep-wake pattern. In sleep, the emotional/soul and 'I'/spirit body free themselves from deep connection within the physical and vital bodies. Your body remains in bed, fully connected to the vital life force which is restoring its strength. Simultaneously, your emotional/soul body processes and discharges its impressions from the day, then fills up anew with vital energy from the sun and other light giving planets, passing it back to replenish your vital body.

During sleep your 'I' spirit connects with your Higher Self, that part of yourself that has not fully incarnated into earthly life. That aspect of your spirit remains untouched and unaffected by events on this earth. Decisions and judgments made are reviewed and when possible, put into right relationship. It is not uncommon to have made a decision the day before, and upon awakening make a change of direction. Or, we may not have any idea of how to proceed and after a great nights' sleep, we awaken clear and determined on the right path to take. These pure 'I' encounters with a Higher Self can radically alter the relationship between persons on earth.

In appropriate rhythmic intervals, the two combed aspects of your fourfold body join and renew themselves, then separate to process and integrate the exchange. This cycle of 'coming and going' occurs four times during a typical nights' sleep. The emotional body contacts the physical body during the REM Phase (rapid eye movement) of sleep. It is giving the vital body energy to restore the physical body while you rest. In this exchange, everything that damaged or strained the body (exhaustion, shock, poison from a heavy metal etc.) is again restored to its original state and is replenished.

In the REM phase dreams usually develop that reflect the activities which occurred during that particular day. If a person is frequently wakened during the REM-phases, the fresh impulses for the vital life body are curtailed. In the long run, sleep deprivation can cause severe health damage at both the physical and psychological level.

People have very individual patterns for the amount of sleep needed. However, it is estimated that approximately one third of our life is spent sleeping. Babies need the most sleep and experience the longest REM-phases. As we age, we sleep for shorter periods of time and the REM-phases diminish in length and intensity. A good deep sleep has a positive and life-enhancing influence on our waking period the following day.

Cycles:

A cycle is an interval of time during which a series of events are regularly repeated in the same order.

Days: Nature warms in the morning while cooling and coming to rest in the evening, and the same is true of us. Cycles of activity and passivity alternate during the course of a day. We tend to be least energetic between 1:30-2:30 PM. Our pulse and breathing slow down at evening, blood pressure drops and our reaction speed slows. Just like the earth sends out its heat into the universe during the day, our body warmth drops during the day, often necessitating the need to keep ourselves warmer in the evening.

While some things diminish, others expand. Our awareness of noise increases at eventide. As the soul releases itself from the intensity of the day's preoccupations, it widens and expands. This is why we are especially contemplative and receptive to 'food for thought' during evening hours. We are more sensitive to beauty and sound; a glorious sunset or evening star thrills our soul, as does a favorite song. Evening is the time when we are most open to new thoughts, questions or differing perspectives. Intuitively we know that a good question always contains something of the answer within it, so evening is an ideal time to ponder a new idea.

Weeks: The week has remarkable rhythm all its own. Rhythm research demonstrates that your soul resonates with each day of the week in a different mood. A certain focus is most easily accomplished on a specific day.

Sunday – Just as rest is needed after activity so we can relax and reflect, it is also needed beforehand, to collect ourselves for decision making. The orchestra conductor, closing his eyes for a moment before raising his baton, is experiencing a little 'Sunday moment'. Sunday rest can invoke inner expectancy and excitement about the things we are thinking of. A Sunday given to rest and reflection provides a source of confidence and strength for initiatives that unfold on successive weekdays. A beginning encapsulates the spirit of the undertaking; *the focus and intentions set on Sunday sets the stage for the following week.*

Monday – On no other day do we encounter as much change as Monday. More than any other day, this requires our openness. The key to right action is the cultivation of the ability for 'active listening'; an open, unprejudiced mood, holding back our own thoughts, ideas and opinions until we have full information from others, makes our own responses richer. The freer we are from prejudice, the more openly we meet and take account of current reality; effectively building new on the old. Growing quiet with focused attention equips us with 'creative spontaneity'—a prepared readiness for action by understanding the situation fully. *Paying specific attention to things outside us is the distinction of Monday.*

Tuesday – The real work begins with dynamism and commitment as action emerges from decisions guided by experience. Here we remove obstructions; hindrances are cleared as we give increasing shape to those Sunday plans. To pursue and realize ones goals involves creating an atmosphere in which mistakes are not seen as regrettable but acknowledged as necessary aspects of development. *Tuesday is an important day to develop a 'culture of mistakes', regarding errors as interesting vs. fatal—it is essential for creative and innovative design.*

Wednesday – The human psyche moves from concentrated activity to an interest in what is happening around us. What have others done and how does it relate to what I have done? Here we pay particular attention to the work and questions of others—a perfect day for meetings. The new ideas we gain enrich our inner life and encourage healthy growth in the project at hand. *Entering into relationships with others is the hallmark of Wednesday.*

Thursday – As the work progresses we suddenly find errors in the work. It shows that some things have been overlooked that could impact further development. Not an error in execution, but one of insight; a key factor has been overlooked. We now take into consideration wider effects and ramifications, much as ecology studies the relationships between organisms and their surroundings. *Thursday is particularly suited for acting in a 'socially ecological' way.*

Friday – The work appears finished: all requirements have been met. Yet it lacks beauty and appeal. Friday is the day we elevate our work into an artistic realm by placing things into a broader context. While proper functioning is required, attractiveness brings acceptance and usage to a higher level. *Friday is the day of the creative human being.*

Saturday- We now look back on the week, not from an analytic evaluation of what went well and what didn't, but rather from a stance of meaning. New relationships and connections between the week's events are noted, tracing deeper-lying causes and motives. These new insights are transformed into personal capacities. *Saturday is the day of maturation and internalization.* We become open for new experiences and ideas—which begin on Sunday.

<u>Seasons:</u> Modern developments have disrupted the natural connection between humans and the rest of nature. Central healing, importing vegetables and fruit from southern lands in the winter, air conditioning in the summer and artificial light detach us from our connections with the seasons. Rhythm research shows that seasonal cycles affect our physical and mental state. Physical performance is greater in summer along with the ability to take in mental stimulation and inspiration from external sources. Our sensory activity fades in autumn as nature comes to rest and the life force of perennial plants and trees withdraw. In the dark of winter we turn our attention from our surroundings back into ourselves in deep introspection.

In spring we immerse ourselves in nature's bountiful diversity in growth and deeper connection with our fellow human beings. In winter's peace and interiority we develop steadfastness. In this season for self-reflection, we ponder our relation with worlds above and around us, creating the foundation for fully engaging again in the dynamic activities of the upcoming spring and summer. Through the human soul, summer and winter join hands. Seeds of autumn and winter start pushing into growth in spring, extending relationships with their surroundings through roots and leaves. In the same way we lay soul-spirit seeds in winter which can become reality in spring and summer.

Transitions:

Transitions involve passing from one state or form to another—these are the most active spiritual moments for us. In the same way that sunrise and sunset offer the greatest wealth of colors in a day, a transitional period offers us special possibilities as well.

Developmental transitions involve moving from one stage of life to another such as exchanging single life for marriage, or shifting from student to fully practicing professional. Each of these major shifts occurs more slowly than the daily rhythms of life. The key to a successful transition is making a 'life-enhancing' choice going forward. What may look like a loss may be a shedding of something that no longer serves us well rather than a setback. To make the best possible decision you may wish to consider the following:

- Does this choice feel right for me?
- Am I interested in where this choice is leading?
- Do I like the people involved?
- Is this choice good for my whole family?
- Does this choice make sense given my stage in life?
- Do I feel morally justified in making this choice?
- Will this choice help me to grow?
- Do I have a chance to be more creative & inspired by what I am about to do?

Focusing on these 'meaning' questions as well as the practical 'who, what, where, when and why' type of issues will help you make a choice that meets both your physical and your spiritual needs. It assures that the *whole* of you is being considered, and honored.

Experiencing the rhythms within daily cycles of life is similar to our sense of time with the minute hand on a clock; we can literally see and experience them. However, deeper transitional change is experienced more like an hour hand; it takes more time to complete, so you only notice it in retrospect. Only in the safe haven of the new way of life does it become clear how lively and active that period of change really was. What may have been a crisis or time of uncertainty is later revealed as a phase of special intensity and great growth.

A major challenge faced by humanity is to learn to experience the changing cycles and seasons of life in harmony and balance, going with the flow without being derailed by it. The dry seasons in life do not last; spring rain will come again. This constant ebb and flow of life stages provides us with the opportunity to continue the human journey, surrounded by ever changing circumstances which continue to grow and deepen us in maturity until the last day of life.

A Living Example of Authentic Connection

Our culture is fixated on the notion of self-esteem; fostering it, having it, and maintaining it—at all costs! We have to succeed, exceeding the performance or expectations of others to have value in our own eyes. Many social relationship and behavioral problems are attributed to 'lack of self-esteem'. A big shift for living a connected and meaningful life is offered in the observations and reflection of a social worker living and working in inner-city New York. After working with disadvantaged youth for many years, she came to believe that the development of self-compassion is more important than self-esteem. This creates the foundation for a culture of learning vs. a culture of blame and competition.

"Over the past decade, research that my colleagues and I have conducted shows that self-compassion is a powerful way to achieve emotional well-being and contentment in our lives, helping us avoid the destructive patterns of fear, negativity, and isolation. More so than self-esteem, the nurturing quality of self-compassion allows us to flourish, to appreciate the beauty and richness of life, even in hard times. When we soothe our agitated minds with self-compassion rather than looking for self-esteem, we're better able to notice what's right as well as what's wrong, so that we can orient ourselves toward that which gives us joy.

Working with disadvantaged youth, we have identified that self-compassion entails three components. First, *self-kindness* requires that we be gentle and understanding with ourselves rather than harshly critical and judgmental. Second, recognition of our *common humanity* fosters feelings of connection with others in the experience of life rather than feeling isolated and alienated by our suffering. Third, *mindfulness*—helps us hold our experience in balanced awareness, rather than ignoring our pain or exaggerating it. We must achieve and combine these three essential elements in order to be truly self-compassionate. Coming from this rather than a competitive perspective, our relationship with others is healthy and life-giving.

Unlike self-esteem, the good feelings of self-compassion do not depend on being special and above average, or on meeting ideal goals. Instead, they come from caring about ourselves—fragile and imperfect yet magnificent as we are. Rather than pitting ourselves against other people in an endless comparison game, we embrace what we share with others and feel more connected and whole in the process. And the good feelings of self-compassion don't go away when we mess up or things go wrong. In fact, self-compassion steps in precisely where self-esteem lets us down—whenever we fail or feel inadequate. Self-compassion is the key to quality relationships with ourselves, with others, with all-of-life."

JoEllen Koerner

Part II
My Canvas: My Biography
Where have you been?

> It takes courage to grow up
> to be who you really are.
>
> E. E. Cummings

_____

Chapter 4

Human Biography:
Patterns of Life

"Always live your
life with your
biography in mind."
Marisha Pessell

WHERE HAVE YOU BEEN? How's it going?
These are questions commonly heard when two
friends meet who have not seen each other for
some time. Like two roads running in many directions, they
now meet at an intersection. Most of the time is spent
catching up on what has been happening in each other's life.
Things which have been long forgotten are recalled once
again—with a common background familiarity. Each asks
questions, makes comments, and shares observations. After
the exchange both go their own way again—but alert in a new
way. In exchanges like this, our past lights up in us in the
moment and new insights are gained, often leading us to
make new decisions or set new objectives going forward.

Our journey through life is an opportunity to look at life
from different perspectives. Each phase is an organ of
perception that enables us to see more of the world and our
self. Every stage presents us with a specific developmental

task that enables us to become more aware of our true, authentic self and our intentions in life. The whole journey is designed for the development of our 'I'; our personal spirit of conscious awareness. In this way we increasingly transform what we have been given into new capacities and higher moral values; we create ourselves anew through our own evolving conscious choices and activities.

When we 'research' our own life, we look at what we have done so far, whom we have met and what our influence upon them and theirs on us has been. We slowly wake up to the fact that we are co-creators of our life, linked together with the whole of creation. In biographical review, we do not need to add anything or change anything, interpret or analyze. *We only need to **see** what is there.* This view often leads to deeper understanding and appreciation for life in general, and ours in particular. A new insight frequently redirects current activities and alters some of our goals, moving us closer to our destiny.

EXPLORING THE LIFE PATH

A biography is more than simply stringing together your life events. Each stage of life has its own quality and specific significance that is important to human development. Every step gradually advances you towards what you want to become during your lifetime, towards your destiny. Two things determine the biography of each person:
  o The universal 'developmental laws' that guide which growth changes will take place during any one phase
  o The specific personal events and situations which you encountered from the outside
Biographical development is systematic growth and change at critical points throughout life that take place in rhythms of seven-year periods. It is your individuality, your unique 'I' spirit, which weaves a unifying thread throughout your life. The older you become, the more aware you are of that 'witness' inside of you that can look back, remembering and

connecting what once appeared to be separate events, while also looking ahead at what is yet to come.

Biography—Stages of Human Development:

Human development follows a 'blueprint for growth'; four cycles made up of 21-year phases that focus on developing different aspects of being human. Each cycle is completed with a crisis that opens up a larger path for the next phase. Growth is always directed towards the end goal—becoming authentic. The life cycle of every living organism goes through periods of growth, equilibrium and then decline. Along with the well understood physical life cycle, your biological, psychological, and spiritual development add important contributions to your maturation.

For the first half of life we test and carry out many of the assumptions, expectations and beliefs that we were taught. Midlife crisis sheds the rules and constraints 'borrowed' from our family and cultural authority. If navigated successfully, the second half of life gifts us with the ability to explore the world on our own terms—bringing all the lessons and insights learned the first half of life into the choices and activities we make going forward. This helps us fulfill our destiny.

4 Cycles of Biographical Development

- **First three 7-year phases (1-21):** Physical & Mental Development—Acquaintance with inner & outer worlds

- **Second three 7-year phases (21-42):** Soul & Psychosocial Development—Acceptance of inner and outer worlds

- **Third three 7-year phases (42-63):** Spirit & 'I' Biography Development—Reflection on inner and outer worlds

- **Final Phase (63 +):** Integration & Contribution—Experiencing oneness of inner and outer worlds

Events and activities of the first half of our life are fairly well established by the structure and 'rules' of society. *After age 42, however, continuing development requires committed self-*

education. At this stage we either maintain status quo in our basic assumptions and life patterns, or we move through 'midlife crises with an awakened sense of who we are and what is possible. That awareness shifts our commitment to our 'true self', prompting us to take bold new steps to redefine our life.

Cycle I- The first twenty-one years (Bodily development)

Your body is genetically determined at conception. You inherit some of the physical features of your parents—along with their emotional characteristics and special interests or talents. Your other three 'bodies' increasingly develop and permeate the physical body during the course of your life until they become fully united—your 'whole' self (at age 21). Human beings are capable of memory from the first experience onward. The thing which is remembered first in a life story is generally decisive for the whole of their destiny.

Indigenous beliefs reference '*7 Generations*', and how much they influence each other. In their world view— you link back three generations (parents, grandparents, great-grandparents) connecting directly with their genetics (physical and biological patterns) and their energy fields (soul-emotional patterns, and spirit- beliefs) . You will influence three generations forward (children, grandchildren, great-grandchildren), extending your genetics and energy field to them. Anything you accomplish physically, mentally, emotionally or spiritually influences them all. Anything unresolved in one generation is passed on as a deeper pattern, making it harder for the next generation to release it—unless healing is done intentionally. True healing includes the resolution and release of intergenerational patterns that are limiting, lifting all 7 generations to higher order. In this belief system, sometimes things occur in our life so that we can heal it for all the generations. This gives noble purpose to our suffering.

> *"Every period of life has its own point, its own purpose. To find it and accept it is one of the most crucial issues relating to the understanding of life."*
> Erich Stern

Phase 1- Physical Growth: Early Childhood 1-7 years; period of fantasy: The human fetus, embedded within the life forces of the mother, learns to independently take on its life functions by the time of birth. For the first several years the infant is still very tender and prone to illness. Physical growth is stronger than at any other period in life. Warmth becomes stabilized and slowly the young child moves out into the world. *At age 3 we have our first experience of 'self': it is no longer 'Jamie wants', but 'I' want!* Safety, nourishment and love are essential until this period ends physically with the eruption of the second set of teeth. This phase establishes a basis for trust going forward. Childhood fantasies, supported and encouraged, establish the foundation for creating a viable social life and career in later years.

Phase 2- Emotional Growth: Youth 7-14 years; period of imaginative life: The rate of physical growth slows downs while the vital rhythmic body increasingly develops in strength, increasing resilience. The energy freed from physical growth now focuses on stimulating the development of our basic emotions and awareness. The child who is encouraged to use their strong imagination will experience the world filled with wonder, beauty and joy. When it is stifled, natural curiosity turns to fear and anger. *At age 9 we begin to withdraw into ourselves more: as our individual feeling life awakens—the beginning of psychological development.* We may notice that we are born into a poor family, or that my feelings are different than my sisters. Here we struggle to come to terms with the difference between 'You' and 'I'. Physically the end of this period is marked by maturing of the facial sinuses; the adult facial characteristics are set. Later this well-developed imagination will foster the capacity for spontaneity and creativity in interpersonal and career-oriented relationships.

Phase 3- Mind Development: Puberty 15-21; adolescent crisis: Once the physical and vital bodies are fully developed, we begin mentally to explore thoroughly the heights and depths of our emotions. *This marks the beginning of soul development, fostering the opportunity to learn to manage one's emotions and to discipline one's focus.* The search for truth begins. Every relationship that is not quite right is noticed; only things genuine are recognized. Book learning is overruled by real experience. What is false at all levels of experience is rejected. This builds the foundation for later spiritual development. The mind increasingly learns how to acquire skill and knowledge that will lead to a career in life.

As we approach the end of this cycle we experience our first maturational challenge: *Adolescent Crisis!* Up until this time the path has been laid out for us by parents and other authority figures. Certain rules and expectations were planted as guidelines for living. The young person increasingly finds themself faced with a universe that is often unfriendly, and not in keeping with the cultural rules of their early childhood. It becomes clear that fantasy and imagination do not create one's reality. Further, they are no longer the center of anyone's world but their own. Disillusioned and confused about their future, working with immature emotions, this upheaval guides the adolescent into the *Search for Truth: "what is the world really like"?*

The main task of adolescence is to stop being one. The issues to be solved if the next stage will be successfully negotiated includes: general emotional maturity; managing sexual interests; successfully leaving the parental home; intellectual maturity; choice of a career; learning to use leisure; constructing a meaningful psychology for living culminating in a moral/ethical orientation towards life; and a self-identity. No wonder it is called a crisis!!

This search for truth—and later for the deeper truth of our own authenticity—is a great one—it fuels our entire life journey. The age of 18.5 has special significance because it is one of three times in our life that we have a clear experience of our path of destiny— *Destiny Opening #1- What occupation do I want to follow while on earth?* It is as if the heavens open a little bit wider and we can recognize inwardly the gifts and inclinations that our ours. The ongoing search for truth is all-encompassing. A balanced access to scientific truth, psychological and spiritual truth lays the foundation for spiritual development in later years: self-education and the search for ideal values becomes a self-initiated adventure.

Under ideal circumstances, the first cycle leads us to experience: 'The world is good', a foundation for a feeling of morality in life. The second seven-year period gives us the basis for aesthetic feelings: 'The world is beautiful.' And if we can question and understand 'truth' in its many forms, we develop the feeling: 'The world is true.' We have learned to display a sense of truth and adopt a critical attitude in life. These foundations provide human beings with the principles of goodness, beauty and truth which belong to all of humanity.

Cycle II- The second twenty-one years (Soul development)

During the next twenty-one year cycle, we learn to develop independently, to establish our own place in the world and give shape to it by taking charge of our health, learning to educate ourselves and balance ourselves both intellectually and emotionally. Finished with formal education, we now must purposefully take the next steps in self-development within a social environment.

Phase 4- Social Development: Early Adulthood 22-28; social establishment : Young adults now begin to look for their own path. They leave the home of parents and childhood friends, wandering out into the world. Events taking place during this phase are oriented around selecting a career, a partner, a home and community in which to raise a family. These choices are strongly determined by feelings, signaling a break from being driven primarily by sentient impulses (sensations, instincts, drives, desires) and cultural conditioning. *This is the beginning of establishing an 'I', self-identity; this awakening personality is the axis around which everything else turns during Cycle II.*

While establishing oneself in the world, this stage also marks the beginning of awareness of an inner world in which drives and instincts begin to be met with a growing mindfulness of responsibility towards other people and social institutions. We struggle with roles; what makes a good parent, employee, spouse? An external life story begins to stand in opposition to our inner life story. If we cannot free ourselves from the rules and prescriptions which were placed on us between ages 7-14, our soul remains caught in its own externally mandated bands and cannot develop further. This inner tension is worked out as we 'try out' our ideas and capacities in private interpersonal relations and life in the work environment. I begin to learn that my viewpoint is not the only correct one. Things can look different from various perspectives and I must learn to look at them from a higher vantage point.

Phase 5- Career Consolidation: Adulthood 29-35; period of objective striving: Until age 28 we are supported by the youthful power of our body, intelligence and enthusiasm—giving flight to our whole being. Towards the end of the twenties, self-awareness and the need for self-expression deepens in response to a crisis of lost physical and emotional capacities. Youth has passed, and emotional waves are less strong. A logical and intellectual approach to life becomes stronger, our ego-filled mind dominating all other activities. 'Now it is time to find out who I really am and what I really can do—my way!'. The initial passion of love has now passed, challenging a marital relationship. We have taken the first evaluation of ourselves and know what we are capable of. We feel a pressing need to take on specific responsibilities and make something of our life; to give shape to, take control over, walk away from something. We are at the zenith of our capacities. With a clearer self-image, we have developed faith in ourselves, believing that things will continue along these lines forever—we are invincible.

Often this hardening of the attitudes, strong ego, and burying oneself in work lays the foundation for later social isolation. Rather than friends, we establish 'relationships', guided by the idea that we are something rather exclusive: 'here I am—and there is the world, ready to be conquered and changed'. This is the most materialistic and self-focused phase in the life cycle. This essential period fully defines our ego-driven relationship with the outer world. Once we experience the fullness of this way of being we begin to feel an emptiness that only a relationship with our inner self can fill.

Many young people pass through a stage of great difficulty between ages 27-35; most typically age 33. The vital life forces are weakened so a crisis of illness is common. Something new has to start at this age. The 'I' has to decide where and how to use its skills and abilities going forward leading to a crisis of talent. The time of inspiration from others is passed so now the 'I' has to start working from its own interior. Many people at this stage have an encounter with a book, a philosophy or a person which guides them to a belief in a Higher Power.

Now the physical body becomes deeply penetrated by our individual self. This gives us strength for external action and our work shows results. We must develop a tolerant attitude of love and respect for all things in our environment to balance the natural egoism of the intellect. This cultivates 'warmth' into our thinking, creating actions and outcomes that are humane. If this is not accomplished a cold and ruthless sensibility prevails. *Either we successfully complete this individualization process, moving on to a more conscious level, or we remain in the unconscious state going forward.*

Phase 6- Mature Adulthood: 35-42; midlife crisis: We are now approaching the mid-point of our earthly life. We gradually have come to feel secure and at home in our work and home environment. We increasingly realize within ourselves what our 'I' with its intentions, beliefs and talents are capable of. We make increasingly creative use of our inner resources, fostering tolerance and respect towards others and we are certain of our path going forward. Accompanying this positive growth is our greatest negative challenge: *we have reached the height of egotism and dictatorship* as well.

This deepening into our self continues by identifying more profoundly with work related tasks and responsibilities. In professional life the priorities may include; the expansion of one's business or realm of work, doing more or better compared with others (competition is high), or making a greater profit. Winning at all costs is the goal.

And then the incomprehensible happens: into this planned and controlled world of assurance, into the middle of this grand scheme, a small doubt creeps in as 'a thief in the night'. Sleepless— events of life are reviewed; small events that went wrong, little irritations, minor disappointments. Suddenly—panic! "Turning 40 and there is nothing new or interesting left. Love my spouse, but after all this time there is nothing novel and new there either". Next morning—it's all gone and life is good. However, with increasing frequency these disruptive thoughts stalk the mind—"I'm not as fast as some of these younger staff members, someone new just came on board, are they going to replace me with her"? And then one fateful day—you are stopped in your tracks by your *second maturational challenge: Midlife Crisis!*

Targets so carefully developed and attained are hollow and empty, void of satisfaction. In this phase your personality and life circumstances gradually come into a real dialogue, accompanied by deepening feelings more mature than earlier emotional waves, increasing your social awareness, and capacity for thoughtful reflection. *This crisis of values marks the beginning of the deepening of one's 'I' consciousness.* The assurance and security of the cycle now ending disappears, opening a way for entering into a completely new and exciting period: the third great cycle of life.

This authenticity crisis invites us to disassemble the illusions which we have about ourselves. Our maturing individuality no longer wants to live for appearances, but for reality. What would remain if I abandoned all of my roles? What are my limits? Where do my capacities and opportunities for life lie? We long to do things, not out of a sense of duty, or because the 'job requires it', but for the sheer love of it. We want to act from the conviction and on the basis of our authentic self.

The age of 37 ushers in 'Destiny Openings#2- Who am I? Here the impulse to make a new start is even stronger than during the first opening at age 18. We experience a strong impulse to leave the past behind us and the urge to adopt new values, new standards. It may mean changing something in our current life that we now have the ability to do, or to make a radical life altering shift.

The soul is shifting from having and doing to being. The having phase is finished: I *have* a wife, a family, a job, a home. But what does that really mean? What have I lost in getting these things: contact with my family, relationships with my children and others, harmony with my inner values? And a real encounter with death is fostered by our physical decline. We reflect more deeply on what we still want to do, what we have neglected to do and what we want to transform into deeds and actions. Or we may gloss over our inner emptiness, avoiding confronting ourselves by escape into materialism, or indulging in alcoholism or other numbing drugs. The way we navigate this crisis has a profound impact on how we experience the second half of life.

We are now in a position to distinguish the important from the non-important, and begin with increasing frequency to sense the spiritual. Relationships with others may deepen as our egotism diminishes, helping perceive the true being of the other person. It ushers in the phase of moving towards mature and fully developed human existence. *From now on development is a matter of seeing what else is inside us, defining a new set of values to guide life from the consciousness of the greater good for all rather than from self-interest.*

The Mid-Life Crisis at Age 42

The forty-second year is a turning point in our life story; an existential crisis of magnitude. While this is a well-known fact, knowledge of things does not free one from living and suffering through them when the time comes. It may occur in the late 30's or well into the next seven-year cycle, but it will be experienced by every human being within this timeframe. People's experience in the following stages will be strongly influenced by what has taken place within them up to this point.

One feels a sense of being trapped in a deep well with no way out. We realize we must fall to the bottom and push off to ascend upwards once again. No one can help us out of this deep pit; we have to give ourselves a hand. Or we sense that we are in a dark tunnel and can't see ahead. But somehow we know there is a light at the other end of it so we keep going. We must answer clarifying questions: What elements inside me can grow or die? What should I revitalize, or encourage to grow? We encounter a spiritual experience of 'crossing the threshold' with growing awareness. When we step out of the darkness we are astounded at the landscape we see. Suddenly the world is filled with images, sounds and colors we were oblivious to previously. We begin to observe and understand this landscape of life from a higher vantage point. *At this time we are finally able to forgive our parents for all their 'perceived failings'.*

This crisis is closely linked to the values and views a person has developed in the preceding phase of Soul Development. It may be delayed by people completely caught up in their external work, careers and success, until well into their late forties, or in mothers/caregivers completely caught up in that role. This prevents the transformation to occur, resulting in increasing dissatisfaction and depression.

The major task of this transitional crisis is to transform our personal, business and life situation from the outside to the inside— achieving inner maturity. At 21 we are partial adults; we become fully mature at age 42. Events in our life have ripened, been transformed and integrated into our personhood. Now we begin to use in increasing measure, the maturity we have acquired for the benefit of others.

Cycle III- The third twenty-one years ('I' Spirit Development)

Fulfillment of the human being—spiritual development (our essential nature) occurs from ages 42-63. Having completed the first two cycles of learning, the human being has reached the 'half-way' point in the biographical journey. During this next cycle a 'second life' can be created. Finding a new value system is not so easy given Western culture's bias for 'intellectual' and 'financial' models of success based on our love for science and technology. However, civilization is on the threshold for exploring new, self-discovered spiritual values. For many of us it is no longer sufficient: to have someone else decide what is good for us; to get what we want at the expense of others; to postpone our own interests and passions while working hard for someone else's. We begin to seek teachers or leaders who can show us new and more conscious ways of being so that we can learn from them and then move on. At the same time (as in all periods of life) we are also teachers for others who are watching us.

Phase 7- Early Aging: 42-49; emotional turmoil & inner searching:
At this point a certain restlessness and dissatisfaction with the course of our life can arise. This mood fosters an opening from which we eventually make a choice; to maintain our current statues, create a different slant on our old life or profession, or open an entirely new way of being. Each choice takes us down a different path as we move from 'stuck' to our 'true destiny'.

Biologically, the vital life force declines in the physical and energy bodies. Digestive juices are no longer as active, making a large steak difficult to digest. Looking in the mirror is discouraging to some as signs of aging such as menopause, shifts in body fat composition, decreasing strength and energy all mark the 'loss' of our old way of being. Psychologically this period is signified by periods of doubt, disorientation, and a tendency towards solutions that are impractical or impossible. Spiritually we wrestle with a sense of emptiness, having lost our old ground and not having found the new.

The discovery of declining vitality, increasing difficulty with which we do and decide things, coupled with a vague dissatisfaction with our own situation, is an attack on our experience of the strongly dominating ego—our sense of self-respect. Individual reactions to this new reality vary enormously. For many who are unprepared, the shocking situation is read as a sign of weakness and all energy is spent pushing back. Pursuing the dynamic career even harder, seeking cosmetic surgery, or taking hormones and drugs, can be accompanied by silencing the discordance through alcohol, sexual adventures, looking for a scapegoat to blame, or sitting passively in front of TV.

While similar to the life choices we made during our adolescent crisis, there is a significant difference this time. In adolescence the crisis occurred during an ascendant life—working with an increase in power and opportunity. This time we are faced with a descendent one, a decrease in opportunity and power coupled with a growing uncertainty about the value of that very same 'life'.

The energy shift unleashes a force for new creativity. We increasingly ask: What might I have buried in gifts, talents, etc. that I could use now? What new impulses and interests am I feeling? We live in a phase where we are still quite active and may develop new personal initiatives, or teach others. We want to communicate something we know, while we are primarily dealing with an age group (21-28) that wants to learn their own lessons. With restraint we wait for younger people to come and ask us. In leadership we can act as a guardian, stepping in only when needed, delegating more tasks to others, while training those who will replace us.

It is during this period of physical decline that the emotional body and 'I' consciousness become further developed and specialized. As physical life and biological forces no longer link up so intensely, the focus of that energy goes increasingly into deepening of our soul and spirit bodies—*the timeline for true inner growth has now been reached.*

Biological decline makes spiritual development possible.

At this time we have the energetic focus, plus lessons from our lived experience of the past 40 years, to foster a wider overview in thinking, greater certainty in judgment, and a deeper sensitivity to our own Self. *We now have all the materials needed to evolve into a stage of wisdom and understanding.*

Phase 8- Mid-Aging: 49-56; redefining ethics & rhythms: With the beginning of spiritual development we encounter a different sense of 'time'. Until now we have only a future and everything is possible. Now, however, that future has acquired a horizon: an end is in sight. Time passes faster and faster, while our past grows longer and longer.

Our will to work grows weaker so we need to make more effort to accomplish the same thing. However, interest in doing things that require judgment utilizing lessons from life experiences increases. Our sense of creativity and spontaneity is enhanced, freeing us from 'ego-imprisonment'. Instead of being driven by assertiveness and the drive for power to achieve a specific outcome, we increasingly find ourselves doing the 'right thing' for the 'right reason' in the 'right way' a 'just the right time'. To our surprise, it takes less effort and gives a more far-reaching outcome than our previous ways of dealing with the world.

As the Mid-life Crisis lessens, we discover whether or not we have found something new. Some individuals cling increasingly to their work. Younger folks become a threat, so they insist on the 'authority' of their position to bring compliance. No longer able to accommodate new situations easily, they cling to the past and idealize their own experience and abilities. Such people are a ball and chain around the leg of their organization.

For those who have come through the crisis with expanded awareness, the early fifties are a true liberation. The horizon expands; new problems of wider significance become apparent. Everyday life becomes more interesting while the distance from little everyday problems increases. There is deeply felt joy in watching and supporting you people grow in their expansionary phase. The result is that this person can give advice and support in a completely new way—and be accepted.

This is also the 'moral and ethical' phase of development. The question arises: What opportunities are there for a better understanding of the world? Can I develop new sense organs to perceive them? We are increasingly less concerned with ourselves than we are with the destiny of humanity. The organ of kindness—the heart—awakens and leads us to suffer and feel sympathy with the whole human race. We become a 'universal father/mother' to the world, and especially to our grandchildren. A new organ for 'listening' is developed; we 'hear' what is going on outside, and grasp the meaning of the event within. This allows us to achieve greater harmony between the rhythms and cycles of the universe and our own.

Phase 9- Mature Aging: 56-63; redefining life purpose & contribution:
The phase from the early to mid-fifties is a harmonious time which ends in still another difficult transition- the _"Aging Crisis"._ New clouds form on the horizon, forcing us to look inward once more. With retirement and death looming ahead we have to identify which values/beliefs are truly our own, and which remain borrowed from others. The question arises: _What are the real fruits of my life on earth?_ We have to prepare for what we still hope to achieve, what needs to be dropped and what we may still be able to finish. There is a growing anxious realization that this is less than we had previously thought. The past passes in review and we see how much we have wasted on trifles—'if only I had more time before me! What, despite my poor choices and actions, might prove to be enduring?'

At age 56 we encounter Destiny Opening #3; How am I going to conclude my life? (you can address these questions at any stage of life—but the momentum to achieve optimal results is greatest when it falls into the designated developmental cycle). Having passed through the refining fire of mid-life crisis, a number of aspects of the human psyche are now available, for the first time, to serve one's life. This opens the door to the greatest clarity and honesty in reflecting on your life, fostering insight and authenticity in the solutions created going forward.

Personal identification with one's own body changes. People engage less in physical activities but are often in a better position to assist, mentor or support others. A great satisfaction— similar to or greater than the joy of one's own personal achievement prior to midlife— is gained by helping others attain their goals.

In a sense, the development of an individual's life has come to a temporary conclusion at the age of 63. Toddler, schoolchild and adolescent make up the youth which gave us a foundation. The second phase of expansion found us engaging in the world of work, friendship and enmity, commanding and obeying, learning what was possible and how to use that insight to grow and mature, both emotionally and spiritually. Clearly finding the edges of our capacity and adopting our own beliefs and values was the gift of the third stage.

We are now poised for a creative and fertile evening of life *if* we have made a commitment to a self-directed inner journey. Crisis and the movement towards death help us transition towards sensing the difference between cleverness and wisdom, between pride and modesty. We can arrive at old age with restraint and acceptance, along with extreme inner capacity that will lead to goodness and peace as we move towards physical decline and dependence on others.

Cycle IV- The final years of life (Body/mind/spirit integration)
After transforming our self from identification with the material world towards an orientation to spirit, we will

increasingly experience the peace and deep satisfaction from a life well-lived. If this shift in focus and detachment is not achieved, our disowned spirit increasingly focuses on the degenerative aspects of our body, and suffering will increase.

Senior citizenship—being ambassadors for the world—is the hallmark of the final life stage. Reflecting on and integrating lessons learned, and applying them with a set of values that transcends material and self-focused ways of being, is aging's crowning glory. This creates the 'wise one' that teaches others by word and example.

There are specific 'developmental tasks' which add depth to our spirit and meaning to life at this time:

o   The ability to disengage from the material life—transform physical forces; we increasingly have less interest in situations and people that merely 'fill our time', choosing to stay home with an interesting book rather than going to a party with people we do not enjoy just to meet a social obligation, etc.
o   The ability to practice independence from one's state of health in regard to feeling well—transforming the soul forces; we experience and acknowledge the shifts in physical body (minor aches and pains, development of chronic condition such as diabetes, etc.) and learn to incorporate those limitations into daily life without being defined—or defining ourselves—by it.
o   To turn to overarching ideals, philosophical and transcendent themes—transformation of spiritual forces; increasingly we are inspired by the great wisdom traditions and reflections on ennobling thoughts which support and inform the wisdom we are realizing as we reflect on life in general, and our life in particular. These 'truths' are now our teacher. They serve as a blessing.

If we achieve these transformations we will develop inner composure and the presence of mind to appreciate every experience of our life. When the memories from our past come to visit, we compassionately see how each event contributed to the development of who we really are. Rather than listening to, or being influenced by the outer world, our inner world becomes a sanctuary filled with original thoughts, ideals and understanding. Choices and decisions are now guided by a mature value system that serves the greater good. These inner qualities and practices provide serenity and a sense of gratitude. This is a personal gain of greater significance than any outer success.

Phase 10- Early Ending Stage: 63-70; integration & stage of wonder:
Once we reach the age of 63, inner development depends less on outer achievement and we allow the delight of wonder to arise in us again. Returning back to the patterns of ages of 0-7, we can now practice qualities which were decisive in our first seven years of life. *We establish a new attitude of awe and wonder* towards nature, our surroundings, or our grandchildren who are developing strong personalities. Looking back to childhood again with our enlarged awareness, we 'see' the issues of the time in the context in which they were lived. We come to understand the challenges and issues facing our parents. *It is a time of identifying the values and gifts granted from our family of origin, and culture of the time, and we develop a deep sense of gratitude.*

We can also allow that child in us to arise in us once more. Unburdened from the responsibilities of earlier life, we often find that we can play in ways never possible before. Patience and focused self-training help us overcome obstacles of the past; we can now radiate true benevolence. When we meet one such elder they give a markedly youthful impression— not so much in the way they look as in their behavior.

Phase 11- Middle Ending Stage: 70-77; cosmic citizen: This period mirrors our second seven-year period of 7-14. The *qualities we acquired through our educational experiences now come into their own.* This does not refer to 'book learning' as much as qualities modeled by earlier role models. If your grandmother was especially generous, you will find yourself manifesting that to your grandchildren and the larger world. The elderly person now has a true capacity to radiate peace, act as a blessing to others and extend sympathy.   Cultivating an attitude of offering support where and when needed offsets an feeling of loneliness and being slighted because of lack of attention. The sanctuary of one's inner world now becomes a very peaceful, warm and nurturing place for the soul.

Phase 12- Final Ending Stage: 77-84+; death by completion: In this phase the youth in us emerges once again. *We engage in a renewed striving for truth.* With death approaching we make a concerted effort to let out bad habits die. We recognize the need to complete things that have a negative energy about them. By approaching ourselves in truth and justice, our deepening and clear conscience requires us to make peace with others and our self.

Now we can see most clearly what we are leaving behind for other generations to follow. *A fruitful life leaves a legacy rich with understanding and generosity of spirit.* Others may live a long time and leave nothing behind, simply vegetating into old age. For a fruitful life we must always be prepared to learn something new—and pass it on—right up to the moment of our death.

We can consciously prepare for death, bringing our life and affairs into order. We put our health and financial affairs into the appropriate legal and ethical structures. Identification of personal issues and relationships that should be celebrated, forgiven or corrected is also important. Planning for our funeral is helpful to loved ones who will carry out those wishes. We may give things of importance to those we wish to bless with the gifts. And, in the end, the unfinished fragments of our life will have been tied up, giving us a death with dignity and joy.

While physical decline is inevitable, the final stages of life make way for the return to the uncluttered mind of a child, only with the wisdom of a fully experienced life. Creativity and imagination return with a depth impossible to young eyes that do not yet see the subtle interconnection of all things. It is important to help older persons' have access to resources and support for the engagement in creative exercises in the fertile evening of their life.

If we consider the achievements of humanity over time, it is the wisdom of old age that holds a set of timeless values that maintains, sustains and elevates life. From the biography of our elders, we can find our way through the complexity and confusion of contemporary society, by understanding their own path into an authentic life. It is here that we will uncover the gifts given to us to enjoy, develop further and then pass on to future generations.

A Living Example of Choosing a Life Path:

Making a decision on life path serves us best when it is made from a deep connection between our innermost being and the outer world in which we live. The challenge is to create an inner life so powerful and profound that it inspires how we live, where we live and how we navigate through life.

Arctic explorer and renowned dog sled guide, Paul Schurke, was interviewed and asked just how he had come to such a life career choice. He stated that when he was 12 years old at a summer camp near Ely, Minnesota, he saw a bear on the opposite shore of the lake from his campground. The sun was setting and he decided then and there that what he wanted was to live by that lake one day. Now he does. When asked to say more, he observed that most people decide what they want to do for a living, and that determines where they live. He went about it the opposite way, he said, has always felt he made the right decision. Consider the connection you have between your inner life and the physical details of where and how you live today. As you review your biography—what patterns do you see?

Chapter 5

My Biography:
The Grand Adventure

"I left the woods for the same reason I went
there. Perhaps it seemed to me that I had several
more lives to live, and could not spare any more
time for that one."
Henry David Thoreau

Having gained an insight into the way life develops,
we are now ready to begin work on our own lived
adventure. A helpful way to gain perspective on
your unique journey is to write it as a story or word picture.
When you see broadly the path taken and the issues
addressed you gain a better understanding of who you are and
the magnificent and unique ways in which you met and
overcame challenges along the way.

This is the story of evolution from Infant to Elder. But to
remember and understand it, memory must serve you well.
By the time we have lived for 40+ years, events and
circumstance lie in vague boxes of memory stored in the
musty attic of our mind. Returning to an earlier time or place
can be facilitated by responding to questions that help us
recall the time of our life and context in which the events
were experienced. The more comprehensive our placement
of event into time and space, the richer the understanding will
be.

A CONTEXT FOR MEMORY

Where were you living when you were twelve years old? What town was it in? Did you live in a house, apartment, housing district? What was your favorite room, place to play, hang out, hide in? Who were you living with; one or both parents, another caregiver, brothers, sisters, extended family? Who were the authority figures in your life at that time; parents and family members, school teachers and church preachers? Our first real memories of our self in relation to others and life gets established at this age.

Draw a blueprint of your home, including those spaces and places that were most important to you. Did you have a pet? Include it. Did you have a bike, a favorite pair of shoes, a book that you reread as if conversing with an old friend? That comfy chair in the living room, or spot by the kitchen table—add all of these things to your picture. Think of favorite foods and odors that bring precious moments to mind—the smell of grandfathers pipe or the aftershave or perfume worn by your parents, the smell of coffee brewing on the stove when you got up to get dressed for school in the morning.

Once you are deeply rooted in that place, review several significant activities that established a core set of beliefs and expectations that served as your guide in life. Recall the rules and messages given to you by the authority figures in your life in regard to the following:

Gender- were there differences between how you and your siblings were treated—based on whether you were first born, last born or somewhere in the middle? Were siblings of the opposite sex treated in a manner different than you were? If so, what were those differences in activities, expectations, privileges, etc.? Do you have a different way of being with members of the opposite sex today that hold some of that same pattern? How does that influence your relationships, personally and at work?

Power- what level of authority was in the roles your parents assumed at home, work, in the community? Were they in positions of power, or working for someone else? What were their attitudes about powerful figures; how did they speak about their parents, bosses, teachers, preachers, government, etc.? Were they respectful, resentful or opinionated based on the issue at hand? How do you feel about authority today, respectful, resentful, or viewed as a helpful associate?

Health- what was your health status growing up; how often were you treated for an illness or injury and how were you treated? Did you get pampered with special privileges or were you told that you were imagining things and had to just keep going? What is your definition of health today and how do you take care of yourself and others? What is your attitude towards pain and suffering? How much empathy and compassion do you have for yourself or others when illness or injury strikes?

Money- what was your financial status at this time? Did you have abundance or scarcity in your life regarding material resources; home and furnishings, clothes and school supplies, gifts at holidays and Christmas? Did you get an allowance or money as needed, or no cash at all? What is your attitude about money today? Do you live with a sense that life is filled with abundance, or does a sense of scarcity haunt you? How does that influence decisions you make about opportunities as they come to you in life?

Work- what occupational roles were filled by your parents throughout your youth? Did the job make the family travel or move frequently? Did it provide opportunities for growth of the whole family? Did it keep one family member 'missing in action' a great deal of the time? Did your parents view work as a privilege, a duty or drudgery? What is your attitude towards work today? How central of a role does it play in your life? How successful are you at achieving work-play balance? Do you live out any of the patterns you experienced in your childhood as it relates to work?

As a youngster, the messages obtained from those in positions of power over us served a very specific purpose. Some assumptions and beliefs will hold true for a lifetime, while others will be outgrown. If held onto unquestioningly, they may limit you later in life. True freedom comes when we can own and respond to our own mind and voice rather than simply reacting out of unexamined rules and guidelines handed down from the past.

RECONSTRUCTING YOUR LIFE STORY

To understand and be understood is one of the great longings of the human heart. There are many biographies of important people. From them we can see decisions and actions that led to moments of greatness or downfall. Also highlighted will be the things sacrificed for a greater gain. While all of these things are instructive, the most important biography is—your own! The more you work on your own life story the more you will come to understand others and the world in which you live.

Reconstructing your life becomes especially fruitful during the second half of life. The first two cycles are very much established by required developmental tasks and the rules of society. However, *after age 42 continued development requires self-motivation and self-direction.* If you truly want to understand yourself and continue to grow towards full authenticity, you are encouraged to create regular intervals of time to work on your own life story in quiet seclusion, or together with a few friends whom you trust. In that way your quest will be enriched by the experiences of others. You will come to see which of the many 'tasks' of life are universal in nature—being experienced by all—and which are unique to your own destiny.

Your true home is not a physical location. It is your mind and the thoughts that accompany you wherever you go. You may move from place to place, but you always take 'I' with you. You can never get a vacation from yourself. *YOU* are the center of your universe....and your life journey is one of increasingly recognizing and becoming aware of who that is.

A common mistake we make in reviewing our life is to look at the growth and decline of our physical body and the 'things' we have in the world; friends, family, jobs, homes, successes and failures. When we define ourselves by outer things—loss and decline are the inevitable outcome. But if you trace the awakening and deepening of your awareness and increasing sense of self-direction—every stage of life is richer than the last. The journey becomes one of growth, and further development until we arrive, in the end, at wholeness; at-one with our authentic self.

In the upcoming exercises, notice how your 'I' awareness shifts and grows; see what prompts you into action and how your decisions are made at various stages of your life. A small baby responds to bodily sensations; crying when it is hungry and fussing when it is wet. The remainder of the time is spent sleeping as the body grows at a rapid rate—all focus and energy is on physical maturity.

Each successive stage has another 'target' for growth and development. The stimulus for our attention, and the combined thoughts/emotions that guide our choices become increasingly more refined and subtle. A mature Elder, in later years, utilizes a wisdom that does not depend on anything external to guide their life. A knowing based on a lifetime of experiences does not need logic or information. Intuitive pattern recognition and imaginative insight sees beyond the obvious. Stripped of old habits and attitudes, we spontaneously and creatively respond in the moment with a fresh solution based on the current situation. *This is the freedom of living an autonomous, awake and meaningful life; the purpose of the journey.*

Your task in biographical mapping is to explore the growth and development of your awareness, identifying the patterns of what focuses your attention and which emotions and intentions guided your choices in each phase. Note how self-awareness evolves into self-direction, and finally into full self-knowing authenticity.

A GUIDE FOR BIOGRAPHICAL REVIEW

(Gratefully adapted from the work of Burkhard, Camps, Lievefgoed & Bamford—see Suggested Reading for more comprehensive works.)

The following Biographical Review Guide is divided into 4 Life Cycles, each comprised of 3 seven-year Phases of Development. It is advised that you take one phase at a time and sit with the questions. Read them through in one setting and let any thoughts or images come to the surface. Jot down notes, a single word or phrase, a comment about a specific event or person, images or memories that surface You may want to find music of that era and play it in the background. Pull out a set of photographs, letters, books, artifacts or gift from someone significant to you at that time in your life; anything that will create a context for your reflective time. Also, while pondering each Phase and Cycle, consider insights gained and how they influence your future.

Cycle #1- Physical Development—Preparation
The primary task of this age (conception – 21) is to grow our body and allow the organs to mature. We do not contribute a great deal to our destiny at this time. Taking and receiving is a characteristic of this stage. Decisions are made by the rules and expectations of others—especially our family of origin. Safety and warmth are the essential characteristics necessary for building a strong emotional base in later years. It is important to understand that there is wide variation in terms of what is considered "normal," driven by a wide variety of genetic, cognitive, physical, family, cultural, nutritional, educational, and environmental factors. Many children will reach some or most of these milestones at

different times from the norm. Human beings grow up and develop at different rates.

First Cycle of Human Development
Focus is on Building a Foundation

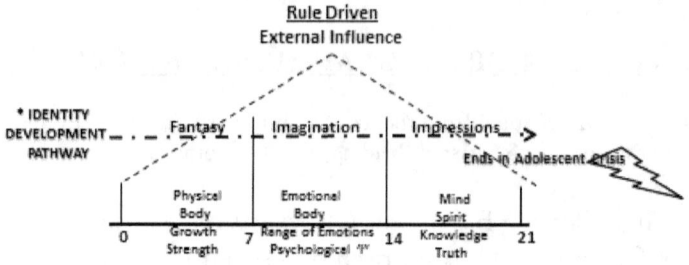

*Most strongly influences emotions and sways decisions

Phase #1- 0-7 The birth process brings together three elements; the individual, their inherited capacities, and the environment in which they are born. Healthy instincts are established. Physical boundaries give security: too many lead to immobility while too few lead to insecurity and restlessness. The soul learns warmth from the emotional environment created by parents. Imagination is fueled by stories and play experiences. Nutrition and hygiene are important. Respected as an individual, _conscious awareness of the self emerges at age 3._ This contributes to preparation for establishing relationships.

- Where do you come from, what was your family name, who were your ancestors, why were you born in this country, town?
- What were you called- any pet names, for how long and by whom?
- What was your birth like- full term, natural, induced, premature, when and where, breastfed, attitudes towards food?

- How old were your parents when you were born- were you wanted as a child?
- Who do you look like- parents, relatives, no one?
- What illnesses did your family have- parents, siblings, were they physical, mental, addictions?
- What is your heritage- nationality, language, faith, occupation of your parents and ancestors?
- Where did you grow up- town, neighborhood, house, landscape, garden, own room, tidy or messy?
- What sort of relationships did you have- with parents, grandparents, siblings, neighbors, classmates?
- Where do you stand in birth order compared to your siblings- youngest, oldest, middle, how many?
- What family habits influenced you- how would you describe the people around you at this time?
- Did you move during this period- how often, where, why?
- What sense-impressions do you recall- smells, colors, touch, sound, nature, garden, animals, land?
- Did you have any pets- what kind, how long, who took care of them, special relationships?
- What activities do you remember- games (indoors or outdoors), camping, trips, holidays, celebrations?
- What peculiarities did you have- tics, fears, rituals or habits, who or what did you imitate?
- What did your world of feelings look like- fears, joys, worries, delights, tantrums, jealousy?
- What formed your religious life- church, prayers, devotion, reverence, love, trust, rituals?
- Did you experience warmth and security- safety, support when ill, injured, forgiven mistaken made?
- What was expected of you- how did you know, what happened if you did not meet it, disciplined, punished, spanked, shamed?
- How did you experience denial- things forbidden, things taken away, things withheld?

- Did you experience the joy of discovery- with family, in nature, at school, with friends, alone?
- What is your first memory- when did you first say 'I' to yourself, what strengths or restrictions come from this era?
- Did you suffer- illnesses, accidents, surgery, inoculations, shocks or losses that could be called 'acts of destiny'?
- Did you develop imagination through play- fairytales, stories, games or toys, TV, books?
- How did you experience school, starting with kindergarten?

Phase #2- 7-14 years of age: This is the period of readiness for school with the unfolding of learning abilities; imagination, repetition and forming of concepts. Capacity for imitation and love for authority figures set habits and norms until- _age 9 when the 'I' awakens feelings of loneliness, loss of certain innocence and a sense of fairness in the emergence of their own values-the beginning of psychological development._ Religious life instills faith and hope, while nature and art offer an aesthetic experience that 'the world is beautiful'. _Twelfth year 'pre-puberty' brings physical and soul changes—beginning soul development._ First serious awareness of; need for one's vocation, knowing that work is required, money is necessary as well as respect for others and their property, sets the notion of boundaries.

- What were your school experiences- when did you start, where did you go, did you like it?
- What type of education did you receive- favorite subjects, most difficult, did you have a good memory?
- What were your study habits- attentive or lazy, good or poor student, relationship with teacher/others?
- How was curiosity fostered- did you get support for the worlds of imagery and imagination from others?
- How did you spend vacations-at home, in nature, on excursions, adventures with neighborhood friends?
- What physical activities did you do- sports, games, contests and other daring acts of courage?

- What duties or chores were yours- what, how often, rewards, what was your responsibility?
- How were your relationships- with parents, siblings, classmates, teachers and authority figures?
- Who was your closest relationship- why, how did your support its growth, how long did it last, why?
- Which people in authority did you fear- why, how do they influence you today?
- What family customs did you have- mealtime, waking and going to bed, birthdays, holidays, illness, successes?
- What behavioral standards were set- which had a positive or negative effect later in life?
- How were punishment and rewards handed out- pocket money, small earnings, spankings, withholding?
- What role did the arts play at home- reading books, music, pictures and art, did you perform any?
- What were your feelings- love/hate, sympathy/jealousy, fear/courage, restless/contented?
- Were you respected- treated fairly, feelings noticed and respected, opinions heard and acknowledged?
- How were your friends treated- brought home, or did you spend more time at their home, no friends?
- How did you dress- what sort of clothes did you have, did you feel beautiful or ugly, self-esteem issues?
- What jobs did you do- any particular chores, which did you like, dislike, why, what did you want to be?

Phase #3- 14-21 years of age: As the physical body and feelings mature, adolescence ushers in the birth of desires, emergence of the personality and sexual development. _This begins the search for 'self' and the quest for truth and knowledge._ There is a struggle between ideals and bodily desires. The circle of friends, groups and clubs play a greater role and family moves into the background. Challenges with adults, parents and teachers are an effort to find one's own selfhood. Authenticity of parents, teachers, religions and the world is questioned. Here we begin to carry responsibility; my deeds have consequences. We are learning to manage outer and inner impressions; what is just, fair, true? Will I be recognized and treated as an adult with equal rights? <u>At 18.5 the first Destiny Opening arrives: the call of a vocation, the value of work.</u> The value of money is also identified. Seduction of drugs and alcohol, along with premature sexuality can hinder growth.

- Where and when did you notice physical changes- how did you deal with them?
- How did you experience your sexual awakening- homosexuality, heterosexuality?
- How strong were your emotions/feelings- did you use drugs, alcohol or have other addictions?
- What was your emotional state- did you experience depression, outbreaks of anger, suicidal thoughts?
- What illnesses did you have- injuries or broken bones, medications—any specific changes around 18?
- What ideals did you entertain- any idols, political, philosophical social interests or involvement—how did you deal with truth?
- What were your interests- how did your schooling progress, what subjects interested you most, least?
- How was your education- easy or difficult time with studies, when did you decide on a career future?
- What were your responsibilities-home, school, at work, in a group, with friends, did your life feel free or forced?
- What were your social activities- girlfriend/boyfriend, friends with shared interests, were you accepted?
- What physical space was yours- your own, shared room, soul space, friends place, private secret space?
- How were you supported- encouraged or opposed by family in life situation and career choices?
- Who were your role models- people who set a good or bad example for you, describe in what way?
- Where would you confide- who could you express yourself to candidly, who understood you, how did you deal with money?

- What were your activities- sports, music, the arts, travel, religious life-were you confirmed or baptized?

Cycle #2- Emotional/Soul Development (21-42)— Expansion

Emotional/Soul Development is the focus of this cycle. Here the major task is self-education and self-development. Our personality, tightly tied to our body in phase 1, now 'comes of age' so we are able to determine and be responsible for the course of our life.

Here we establish a family, a home, and a career. We develop social bonds and connections, taking our cues from other people. We experience a multitude of emotions, confrontation, love, enthusiasm, antagonism from others. *We must learn to live with our feelings and bring our ego under control.* Through all these existential battles our soul is refined and *we achieve psychological and emotional maturity.* Generative and degenerative forces are balanced at this point. We develop ourselves as 'individuals' in the world; we are now grown up. Give and take marks the joys and struggles of

Second Cycle of Human Development
Focus is on Maturing the Emotional Soul

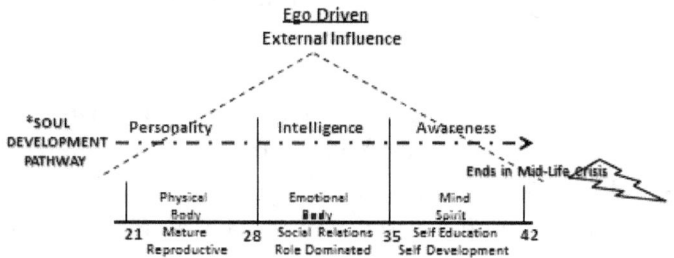

*Most strongly influences emotions and sways decisions

Phase #4- 21-28 years of age: Age 21 marks the period where the personality is striving for autonomy and self-awareness while the emotional soul is influenced most strongly by the senses- mirroring the first seven years of life. *An identity crisis occurs as we try to find our own place in the world- the birth of the 'I'.*

New experiences, adventure and travel (both inner and outer) are sought. Insecurity is part of this phase as the soul is reliant on the outside world. Multiple roles are taken on; there is a danger that they can stifle or immobilize us. Natural enthusiasm is high and ideals know no boundaries, causing frequent mood swings. My point of view is the right one! Others opinion begins to matter and professional partnerships and groups of similar interest are sought. There is a battle for personal freedom and independence from parental influence. *Age 27-28 brings a crisis regarding talent; we now recognize our gifts and a vocation is established.* In emotional and romantic relationships we look for someone who completes us. The relationship is mostly full of expectations, demands, frustrations and dependency.

- How did you feel about life at age 21- did you go through a crisis at this time?
- When did you start to live away from your family- when did you become financially independent?
- Were you following the right course of study or career path- did you earn money during school?
- Did you live with someone or live alone- how did you choose a partner?
- Did you start a family- have children, how many, what was your relationship with them?
- How would you characterize your lifestyle- what roles did you take upon yourself— any changes around 27-28?
- Did your roles weigh upon you- on the family, or could you develop your personality?
- What were your emotional moods-how would others evaluate you, were you fearful about life, strong feelings-anger, guilt?
- Were you part of communities- living communities, work groups, teams, cliques, any sports, hobbies etc..?

- How did outer experiences affect you- strengthening or weakening—what was your view of life & world at this time?
- Did you enjoy life- outside work, travel, what were your interests, did you meet other people?
- What were your work ambitions- were you able to put your ideals into practice with success?
- Did you have a mentor or good supervisor in work or were you self -taught- did your work satisfy you?
- What picture did others have of you- you have of yourself, which inner values did you maintain in work/marriage?
- What tasks did you enjoy- which ones did you reluctantly undertake?
- Did you experience your own limitations- what were they, did new capacities show themselves?
- Were you more introverted or extroverted- more active or passive, what frustrated you, any psychic crisis at this time?

Phase #5- 28-35 years of age: This is the period of partnership between the deepening mind (we identify with ideas, ideals and externally-generated thoughts) and the intelligent soul (emotional responds more strongly to thoughts and expectations than the senses); it mirrors the second 7 year period of life. _The primary questions are about how the world is organized, and how one can organize their self in the world._ This concerns both personal and family life, and professional occupation. Talents and gifts need to be managed from within rather than through the direction and opinions of others. _The 'I' deepens as an inner space is forming to serve as the foundation of one's existence._ Experience becomes the security of life: identity is tied to role in life and tasks accomplished.

This is the most deeply incarnated point in life with physical and ego-strength at their greatest. Organization and planning become visible and work and worth are recognized. Previous lack of belief is left behind and a new spiritual awareness takes place. Strength and capacities give a feeling of security. Thinking has become ordered and intellectual thought is beginning to add heart warmth and understanding to it. Personal mission and motivation become the guiding principle. In a personal partnership, inner searching seeks more individuality and independence. This process of individuation is painful in the relationship; a separation of emotions occurs within the soul, but not necessarily a divorce. Each partner becomes more whole- but not perfect. The relationship ends or a new form of love and companionship is created between two who have become independent and now join together as equals.

- Who were the most important people in your life at this time?
- How was your family life- did you find your place in it without being stifled, without stifling others?
- How was your relationship with your partner, children, parents, friends, did you love your partner- was love returned?
- How did you organize your professional life- any ideas brought to fruition, which ones, right job, coworkers, place, tasks?
- Was there a rhythm at work- balance between work and family life, active social life, sports, art etc.?
- Were there meaningful occurrences at this time- insights, intuitive flashes, what were they—special experiences 30-33?
- Were you able to express your feelings- with clarity and objectivity; any illnesses, psychic crisis or accidents?
- How were your relationships with men and women?
- Did you form inner space within yourself- or did you live entirely outward- what lived in you as inner truth?
- Where were situations of conflict- how did you deal with your compulsions and addictions?
- Did you still receive assistance from parents- the state?
- Did you own a home- in what did you invest, did you have debts?

- How did this seven-year period affect your later life?

Phase #6- 35-42 years of age: The 'I' identity is now influenced by own awareness rather than the input from others, mirroring the awakening adolescent phase of our life. Our emotions are inspired by inner feelings rather than externally imposed ones; inner generated awareness and feelings join forces. Physical regeneration is more difficult but the decline of the body frees the life forces to focus on the development of consciousness. An awareness of death arises; what will I take with me after death? Emptiness is found in the routines of work and family. Activities to blot out the hollow feelings may include drugs, sex, more possessions. Or courage prevails and *the pursuit of self-knowledge begins.* Questions about potentials and limitations are combined with acknowledgment of personal failures and the lessons learned from them.

At this time of re-evaluation, outworn values are left behind and new ones adopted. *Life experience rather than intelligence now becomes the teacher.* Destiny becomes more visible. At age 37 the second Destiny Opening causes an authenticity crisis *as roles are shed and a more spontaneous stance is taken towards life.* This shift fosters efforts to transform our current reality into something new; a possible career change or new tasks or responsibilities. *The excuse of blaming parents for all personal failures comes to an end.* A series of crisis, challenges, pain or separation occur, sharpening social skills. In personal relationship there is a danger that each partner goes their own way; creating a distance between them. Dialogue is essential to uncover new and shared values and aims. Love becomes more authentic, no longer based on rules or obligations. The essence of the other is now made visible and the relationship can deepen.

- Did anything special occur around the 35th-37th year?
- When did you notice a lessening of vitality- did you know your own limitations, potentials?

81

- Were you subject to particular anxieties- fear of death, feeling you would not live much longer, etc.?
- Did you accept challenges- what did you find easy, difficult?
- Did you experience inner emptiness- how did you deal with it?
- What picture did others have of you- you have of yourself, was there a gap, how did you notice it, close it, or did you?
- Did you experience a sense of impostor, what happened then?
- Were you able to reconcile yourself with your parents- did you undertake a self re-evaluation?
- Did changes take place in work or family life as a result of your new values- what did you do?
- Were you on the path to bring your guiding principle(s) to fruition?
- How was your situation- physical space, soul space, spiritual space, home, work, friendship?
- How was your situation with your partner- empty void or new deepening relationship?
- What was your status in the work environment- how did you deal with routine matters, with changes in the workplace?
- What value did money hold for you- in relation to work?
- What was your attitude regarding death- pain, anxiety; did you find spiritual values, which ones?
- Were you faithful to your new principles and ideals- what did the world receive through you?
- What sort of relationship did you have with others- how did you work with family, groups, others?
- Did you have any particular illnesses- psychological crisis, accidents, addictions, workaholism?

Cycle #3- Spiritual 'I' Mind Development—Reflection.
Having completed the first two cycles of learning, we reach the half-way point of the journey. Going forward, the

primary task of this age (42-63) is to create a 'second life', adopting a new value system that is our own. We begin the search for true self-identity and authenticity.

Third Cycle of Human Development
Focus is on Expansion of Mind/ 'I' Spirit

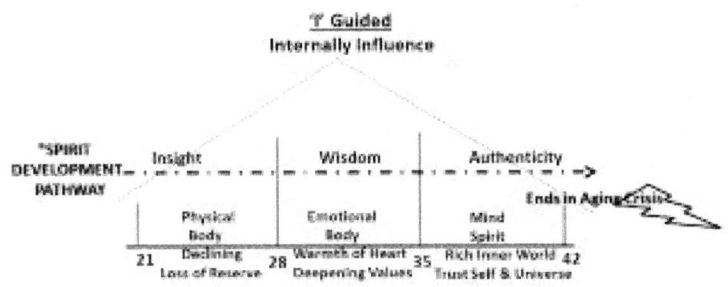

*Most strongly influences emotions and sways decisions

Phase #7- 42-49 years of age: An existential crisis of existence begins. It feels like the ground under our feet is disappearing with thoughts such as "It's too late", "I am getting bogged down" or "Something is wrong—I just can't get a handle on myself anymore!". Towards the end of this period, female menopause begins; the old life has ended. When the crisis is over, there is a deep feeling of completion: the end of hierarchical influences has occurred. One comes out of this phase transformed, or in some instances serious illness and even death can occur.

Our varied life experiences have matured into the pattern recognition of intuition. It begins to merge with our 'I' mind, providing insight to our awareness. Thoughts, emotions and actions are now cultivated from a broader view of life. A deeper understanding of the relationship between things seen and unseen are available to us as we observe life and choose our responses to it. Altruism begins (or one becomes a tyrant). We can now observe drama in the workplace without being drawn into it; we stay emotionally balanced. We find a new courage for the deeds to be done and a more inclusive style of leadership emerges. Good looks fade but we are more comfortable in our skin as the life forces continue to loosen. Those who fear aging often seek a second adolescence; sports, drugs, excesses and distractions.

- What sort of inner and outer changes did you experience at 42?
- Did you find yourself in crisis- what caused it, did you face it, with fear, courage, or both?
- Did you feel supported- or alone, how was your relationship with your partner, children, parents
- How did you deal with diminishing good looks- strength, sports capacity, physical ability?
- Did you fall in love again- how did you deal with this?
- Did you feel threatened by younger people at work- did you change the way you worked?
- Did you develop a new form of leadership- pass on what you know, taking care of others who follow?
- Did you experience emptiness as your children grew up- did you try to bind them to you?
- Were you competitive with younger colleagues- with your children?
- Did you feel creative- were you able to achieve your life goals or were you paralyze
- Were you able to live with new values- could you reconcile your new inner truth with your outer reality?
- What habits did you need to change- if you were to continue to develop what did you need to change?
- Were you able to give up everything you had done/made to this point if necessary?
- Did you experience authenticity in your actions or continue to act out of norms or follow a specific role?
- Did you take on, or let go of, any social tasks, hobbies, activities, responsibilities?
- Were you aware of any special changes taking place around the age of 48?
- What illnesses or crisis did you go through-accidents, drugs, medications, alcohol, etc.?

Phase #8- 49-56 years of age: This period, following the turbulence of the past two phases, brings us to increasing selflessness, contentment and harmony, and a state of wisdom. The strong reasoning of our intelligence deepens, expanding into inspiration in the moment. Thinking gives way to wisdom, (thought warmed with the heart). This new phase of wisdom is where information and knowledge become practical as a result of our many and varied life experiences. We pay more attention to our authentic inner voice. Greater discernment is made regarding which questions and tasks coming to us from the outer world we want to engage with. We increasingly realize that our life has taken place, so now we turn towards the larger tasks of humanity. *This is the moral/ethical phase of our journey.* Life and all its endeavors come into harmony with our true inner self. We feel a responsibility towards younger generations. With humility and graciousness we delegate our work to those personalities with leadership qualities which we had trained in the previous seven-year period.

A new life rhythm needs to be found; a shift in values guides this redefinition of who we are and what we are meant to do next. Changes take place in our inner world as our spiritual and aesthetic feelings and understandings deepen. Life is transformed into a living blessing. Age 56 ushers in the final <u>Destiny Opening: what do I want to leave behind?</u> Male andropause takes place. Many careerists and professionals find themselves at the peak of their career. Those unable to free up from old situations, family conditioning and expectations, may pressure children or work colleagues to continue their work. This can interfere with healthy intergenerational or organizational relationships. We either move gracefully into the next stage of our life or remain in old situations, losing our effectiveness, and often, the legacy we would have left behind had we made the exit at this more ideal time.

- How did the transition to this new way of being unfold during your 49th year?
- How did you find a new life rhythm- were you flexible, rising to new challenges, or immobile, stuck?

- How did you bring the wisdom of your life experience to others- did you teach or instruct, write, speak?
- Did you have the ability to give your strengths to others while leaving them free in their own right?
- How did you get along with younger people- your children, grandchildren?
- What universal human tasks came to you, or did you take up in a new way?
- What new aims, ideals and interests were you able to take up- what were the new accomplishments?
- Did you feel in harmony with your morals and ethics- which thoughts or habits did you change?
- Did you have any spiritual or religious strivings?
- Did you lead a harmonious and balanced life- was something missing, how did you address that?
- How did you deal with your sexuality?
- How did age 55 ½ affect you (Destiny Opening)- were there inner or outer changes, what were they?
- What illnesses, psychological or other crisis, accidents did you have – drugs, meds, additions?
- If a woman, when and how did menopause take place- what changed after that, how was it dealt with?
- In what way did this seven-year period affect the later years in your life?

Phase #9- 56-63 years of age: Intuition and insight now merge more deeply with the wisdom brought to the moment, fostering mindful living. While the physical body becomes more inflexible, the inner human becomes increasingly spiritual and fluid in nature. We frequently turn inward, pondering philosophical life questions: Have I fulfilled my spiritual mission, my life's motivation? What is left that I am to do? What will I take with me into death, is another theme of thought. Looking back is challenging as one sees more clearly mistakes and misjudgments. *Self-criticism and renunciation are the norm--the existential crisis of aging.* How we truthfully come to terms with all that we have done is central to the final stage of life (more in the chapter on aging).

Inner experiences of dying make space for cultivating our inner world after the 63rd year. Externally, we increasingly step into the background, staying close if we are needed. We give our positions of power and authority to younger ones with the energy and social alignment to succeed in a way congruent with the needs of a changing society.

We begin to replace our 12 mature senses with 12 virtues—the foundation of moral character. Virtues are not something we can learn, they are something we become: peaceful, generous, trustworthy, kind, etc. Bitterness, feelings of guilt and frustration may poison our life and the life of others if inner work is not tended to consciously. The loss of a partner may call us to new tasks. **It is possible for us to bypass the living of our own life going forward by existing in the illusory life brought to us by mass media and social norms.**

Retirement will have the effect of threat or liberation. A false sense of security can be created through pensions, insurances etc., taking the place of inner security.

- How did you experience the transition from the 55th-56th year- any crisis, inner or outer changes?

- How did your sense organs function- did you care for your health, in what ways?
- What was the state of your memory- what exercises did you do to maintain or improve your memory?
  - o What was the state of your physical mobility- what exercises did you do to remain mobile?
  - Did you suffer from sorrows, disappointments, frustrations- what were they, how did you cope?
  - What purpose did you see for your life at this point- how did you achieve your life ambitions?
  - What would like to develop in the future- what does your future plan look like?

- How did you deal with bereavement- did you grieve and go on living, or did you quit living?
- Do you enjoy learning new things- what interests, activities, hobbies, books, classes did you pursue?
- Was it possible for you to finance the coming years of your life- did you organize estate administration?
- What was the state of your relationships- partner, children, grandchildren, living parents, friends, other?
- How was your relationship to younger generations- what was your attitude about social change etc.?
- What ties did you still have remaining to your life- what things still need to be regulated, reconciled?
- How did you envision retirement- where, how, with whom, when, etc.?
- Did you suffer from any illnesses, operations, accidents or addictions- use of medications and drugs?

Cycle #4- Body/Mind/Spirit Integration —Completion

The primary task of this final stage (64++) is to detach from the outer world and increasingly deepen and live with peace and gratitude in the inner oasis of our being. Activities which 'give back' to society are sought, accompanied by the deep satisfaction of a life well-lived.

Forth Cycle of Human Development
Focus is on Integration

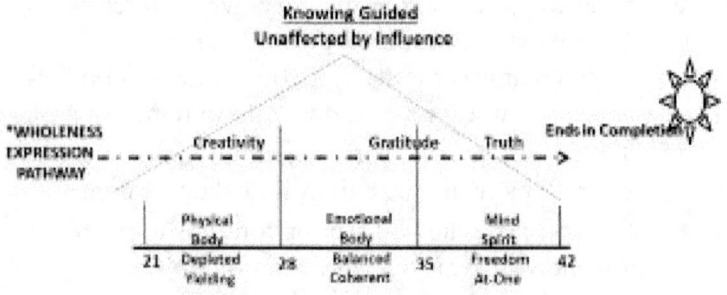

Phase #10- 64-70 years of age:: Inner development depends less on outer achievement; the mirror of early childhood reappears. A return to ages 0-7, we develop a new sense of wonder, awe and delight towards nature, our surroundings and our grandchildren. Curiosity is heightened and the discovery of hidden or long-neglected interests and talents is resurrected. *Creativity and playfulness is at an all-time high.* There is more contentment being alone or with nature than engaging in meaningless social activities.

Phase #11- 70-77 years of age:: The age of the Senior Citizen mirrors the period of 7-14 earlier in your life. Qualities acquired in the education of one's youth come into their own. Not only academic skills, but life skills modeled by parents, grandparents, and the culture of the time resurface, enriching our understanding of, and appreciation for, the countless blessings of our youth. *A deep sense of gratitude and generosity fills our being.*

Phase #12- 77-84++ years of age:: This phase reflects the period of adolescence in earlier life. A final search for truth is undertaken. Impending death kindles a desire to complete all negative elements remaining in our life. A concerted effort is made to let bad habits die, repair damaged relationships or situations, and celebrate the people, places and events that contributed richly to the life journey. Putting personal, financial and emotional affairs in order facilitates a 'death by completion'.

The following series of questions can be applied to any of the final three phases of life.

- What do I still want to learn and do in the future- interests, abilities, capacities remaining?
- What new dimensions of awareness and understanding are opening for me- personal, spiritual?
- What are my predominant emotions- gratitude, thankfulness, generosity, fear, anger, resentment?
- How do I succeed in preserving some of the gifts, insights from my childhood for other generations?

- What kind of social environment do I enjoy- being alone, in the company of others- who and how much?
- How will I live- with spouse, alone, with family, a retirement home or communal group?
- What is your relationship with your children and grandchildren- causal, close, distant, strained?
- What do you enjoy most of all- travel, reading, physical activities, mental activities, solitude and silence?
- What annoys you most of all- things, weather, other people, politics, noise, traffic, etc.?
- What distresses you- is there anything you would like to change?
- Who do you have something to say to- thank you, I am sorry, etc.?
- What would help you feel that you have 'completed' your destiny assignment- how can you finish it?

EXPLORING YOUR PATTERNS

As you work through each Phase, you will start to identify certain patterns that reoccur. Clarity about these tendencies is extremely helpful at times of transition in your life.

#1- Recurring Life Patterns: You may uncover a tendency to be drawn to certain things, or a theme that repeats itself in cyclical fashion. You may see certain relationship issues that keep showing up through the years. To become more clear about them consider some of the following questions:

- What is the greatest challenge in your life that has become clear to you as it has been with you since your earliest memory?
- Are there situations in your life that keep repeating themselves over and over?
- What do you find difficult, irrespective of age- where are the challenges?
- What gifts do you have that served you well in every age- how did you cultivate them?

- What 'old patterns' do you need to eliminate from your life so 'new growth' can occur?
- What is your guiding principle in life, a golden thread running through it?
- Are you on a path that will fulfill your deepest life desires and your destiny?

#2- Transitional Stages: A transitional stage is one which fundamentally changes things in irreversible fashion; moving from single to married, a mid-life career shift, having children, a life-altering illness, changing home or residence. Each of these requires deep consideration of the physical, mental, emotional and spiritual dimensions of our life. Revisit questions in Chapter 3, 38-39. Focusing on these 'meaning' questions as well as the practical 'who, what, where, when and why' type of issues will help you make a choice that meets both your physical and your spiritual needs. It assures that the *whole* of you is being considered, and honored.

#3- Career Changes -Especially after 30: As we approach the second-half of life, a common challenge is the questions 'what should I be doing with my life?' In order to discern your vocational path, consider some of the following::

- Do you feel that you have found your right career- do you enjoy it, are you in the right place?
- Have you found the right people to work with- are you in the right relationship with them?
- Are you doing what seems right- does it correspond with your values, qualities and abilities?
- In which area does your interests lie- research, overseeing, planning, organizing, enterprise, supporting, fostering, caring, renewing, brining into action, conserving, keeping records?
- What future possibilities exist in your current career?
- Aside from developing your career possibilities, do you have the opportunity to develop the human side of your being within the work setting?

- What are the challenges in this current position?
- Do you have the opportunity to use your full potential?
- Do you find it easy to be with superiors and subordinates? Why? Where do you find difficulties?
- What do you enjoy doing?
- What are you unwilling to do?

Once you have an understanding of how your life has developed over time, mapping events into specific configurations will give you insight into the development of your soul and your spirit. Because the second half of life mirror's the first half, by laying out the significant moments of your life—side by side—you will see how and where those events occur. Once understood, you can respond to the cyclical events with insight and clarity—shifting things in your biography going forward in a way that enhances the quality and direction of your life. This is explored in the next chapter.

A Living Example of Envisioning the Future:
By using our imagination and our intentions, we can look ahead in time and practice various scenarios about what it might look like. Scenario planning is not just a strategic planning tool for large corporations seeking a successful future. It can also give us insight into what would be most meaningful for us. A sixty year old CEO shared his experience at a retirement party.

'About thirty years ago, lying on my back staring at the sky in a park in downtown Toronto, I began to wonder what my life would be like when I reached the age of 67. I pictured myself as being wiser, more balanced and self-aware than I was then at the age of twenty-six. I pictured myself as having gotten most of what I wanted to get out of life. I was living in a simple home with big windows back in the woods near a lake. I imagined that my average day included both hard physical work and deep rest.

I then imagined a conversation with this person I hoped to become. I walked into his living room and sat down. The room was quiet. I asked him a question. He turned, looked over his shoulder out the window, got up and left without saying anything. He walked down to the shore of the lake, got in his canoe, and went out for an early evening paddle.

After thinking awhile about this, I concluded that what he was saying to me was that a lot of the things that I thought were important really weren't, including the question I had just asked. Many of the things that were preoccupying me in my mid-twenties had little to do with what would eventually prove to be important in my life. What was important, my future self was saying, was to orient myself and my life around quiet beauty, natural beauty. When I've deviated from that life path, the ultimate result has invariably been adverse.

I've often since turned to that imaginary future self for advice. Many times the feedback has been tough to take. It has directed me in directions I didn't want to go and so I've often rejected the advice. I've sometimes thought of my future self as Mr. Kill Joy. "I know you. You always opt for the route that is the least fun. You are kind of dull." In retrospect, I was wrong. Following the advice offered, while it would have meant some missed fun, would have generally meant avoiding wasted effort and heartache. On the other hand, a balanced life needs fun too.

Building and nurturing a relationship with mySelf is important work. And when I listen to what I really know, I keep myself honest—and out of trouble. Maybe I should become my own best friend!

Chapter 6

Understanding Biography:
My Life's Meaning

> "To be what we are, and
> to become what we are
> capable of becoming, is
> the only end of life."
> Robert Louis Stevenson

O ur journey through life gives us an opportunity to look at the world from various perspectives. Each age and stage gives us a different set of experiences, developmental tasks and the viewpoint appropriate to navigate that terrain. It also gives us an increasingly broader view of the world and who we are. We increasingly awaken to our authentic self; our 'I'. The potential within our innermost self continues to grow throughout each phase and its varied activities. We increasingly take lessons learned and transform them into new capacities of higher senses, spirit and moral values. In every phase and stage of life we create ourselves anew through our own conscious activity.

In the essence of all living things resides the desire to connect with a Higher Spirit. Working consciously with the material in our lives is a pathway to discovering ourselves at this deeper and more subtle level. It is a path of heart that arises from our feelings and intentions. When we can see beyond the physical boundaries of our daily life into a moment-in-time where past and future coexist, a sense of our destiny is felt. This is the guide that brings us to our life purpose and meaningful existence. Only then are we truly human.

MAPPING YOUR LIFE STORY

If you completed the activities in the previous chapter, the story you created is an excellent tool to use throughout the biography maps offered in this chapter. Several guiding principles in biographical review are helpful to maximize the effectiveness of the process:

o   It is not easy to look objectively at another person. Usually our first thought is of what good or bad the other has done to us in the past. Allow that thought to pass through you, and then try to look at that person with empathy. At some point we begin to look at teachers, friends, all those who have helped us as well as those who injured us (who from a certain point of view were even more instrumental in our growth and development) simply as players in our life drama. The ability to picture ourselves and others without love or hate, helps us see everyone and everything (including ourselves) more clearly and more fully. This process will develop our higher senses.

o   Looking at a single event does not always show relationships over time. It is helpful to explore a situation, and the feelings it created. Then move forward in your biography and see where and how that pattern or emotional response continued to be replayed. Often we react to a situation with a habit learned earlier in time. Identifying and disconnecting from these habitual reactions is central to developing the true freedom to simply show up later in life and live authentically in the moment.

o   While it is important to strive for accuracy, more important is to remember the impact of the event and the meaning and insights you acquired as a result of it.

Panoramic Life Review:

There are numerous ways to approach your life story, depending on your preference. To create a broad review of your entire life. write down the significant events and then later place them into a map. Highlight the moments that you consider essential for your self-understanding. Using a blank sheet of paper, create a Linear Life Review Matrix, starting with the year of your birth. Map every 'developmental crisis'; I started grade school at age 6, graduated from high school at age 18 etc. Once you have finished with the expected ages and stages of life, return to the beginning and identify each 'situational crisis'; at age 5 my father died, surgery at age 34. At age 57 I took up painting once again, etc. Note every event that stands out in your memory. (If you would like to go deeper, refer to the questions in Chapter 5).

Linear Life Review Matrix

Stage #1-Physical Development	*Stage #2- Soul Development*	*Stage #3- Spirit-'I' Development*
Phase 1: 0-7 years	**Phase 4: 21-28**	**Phase 7: 43-59**
– 1-	– 22	– 43
– 2	– 23	– 44
– 3	– 24	– 45
– 4	– 25	– 46
– 5	– 26	– 47
– 6	– 27	– 48
– 7	– 28	– 49
Phase 2: 7-14	**Phase 5: 28-35**	**Phase 8: 49-56**
– 8	– 29	– 50
– 9	– 30	– 51
– 10	– 31	– 52
– 11	– 32	– 53
– 12	– 33	– 54
– 13	– 34	– 55
– 14	– 35	– 56
Phase 3: 14-21	**Phase 6: 35-42**	**Phase 9: 56-70**
– 15	– 36	– 57
– 16	– 37	– 58
– 17	– 38	– 59
– 18	– 39	– 60
– 19	– 40	– 61
– 20	– 41	– 62
– 21	– 42	– 63

Writing down the events is a therapeutic act in itself. It helps us form and order our thoughts. If we maintain a diary, looking back several years is always a surprise as there are many things we cannot see until we look at them from a distance. It is advisable to write your selected moments in the form of a diary. The key events in life can be selected and placed into the life review matrix.

You may wish to begin with a single event. It is helpful to place it in the month/day/time and space in which it occurred. Try to visualize the whole scene, everything that occurred in as much detail as possible.

Recall your age, how you were dressed, what your hair style was, where you were living at the time. Describe in detail the environment where the event took place: street, room, garden, school, pictures on the wall, smells and noises, who else was with you. Make the image so clear and alive that you are able to feel the experience as if you were there once again.

Now describe the feelings you experienced during the event. Don't forget that you are the observer to the scene— do not get hooked back into any drama from an insiders' perspective as much as possible because it will color your objectivity. If the situation still is emotionally charged or unresolved, you can work with it in other mediums such as expressions in art such as clay, painting or drawing, or journaling. This is a therapeutic way to bring healing to the situation. Once you have gotten clear about what happened, identify how you would have liked it to end. Explore what would have been different, what you would have learned and what you would have missed. Remember the Rule of Unintended Consequences: in every positive situation there is an outcome that was not as helpful as it may have been. And, in each difficult experience there is usually some redeeming quality or insight that you would not have if the experience had not been yours. Look for those elements. If your relationship to the situation has changed since it first occurred, note what has shifted and what that represents as growth for you.

Knowing the developmental tasks of that phase, explore how it influenced your impressions and actions. Identify if your experience was one that most people of that age/stage go through, or if it was uniquely part of your biography. Then question: Has the situation occurred before in my life or was it a single event? This objectifies your own biography.

Rather than a single event, you may choose one event from each 7-year period to work with if you want to look more broadly at your life journey. Or you may also wish to work on an emotional level. Study the situations you identified as significant and note the emotions that each event evoked. Then give each 7-year period a different color that represents how you were feeling during that period. (This is especially helpful later in working with mirror images). Reviewing your list, note what emotions the various periods of your life held . A woman looks back on her youth, remembering her need to step into the mother role early as her mother passed when she was 6. Her life had been a dutiful one, devoid of a carefree childhood. She watches her daughter, full of life, with unlimited ability to play and be free. At a deep level she feels some jealousy and resentment. How do we handle such honest feelings?

Which events or themes are repeated throughout your life story; i.e. 'I change jobs every 3-4 years, why is that'? or 'I keep falling in love with men who are trouble. Is it due to me or the men"? Ask yourself if you want to change the situation or is it something that you cherish and want to keep repeating?

If you can complete this process with several others, it is very beneficial to share your story with them. It is important to recreate the key elements in your life as you share your experience. Only tell those things you are comfortable sharing voluntarily. Others are invited to ask questions to help clarify and deepen the details. As you tell your story, it will bring out hidden memories and feelings of others in the group. Each one awakens inwardly, gaining a better insight into their own life.

Many people talk about what they have missed in life, but basically they have not missed anything. For while they were studying, or working to support the family, etc., they replaced what they think they missed with something else of vital importance. The art of living is to pay attention to the opportunities that come our way in life and determine if we have used them appropriately. Are we happy with the outcome? If in truth there is something to 'catch up on', the important thing is how we do it.

SOUL DEVELOPMENT—SECOND LIFE CYCLE

Soul development is the primary task of the second round of life. Once the first cycle is finished, our life focus and vital energy pour into development of the emotional body. Biographical Mirroring helps us explore how the first stage of life reappears during the second and third, giving us an opportunity to re-experience patterns, learn valuable lessons and grow in capacity and discernment.

Temperament is a composite of the natural tendencies we are born with, the unique pattern of thinking, behaving and reacting that dominate the first life cycle. *Personality* becomes the main driver as we move into the second series. It is the blend of our natural tendencies and the social world in which we live—a face we show the outer world. In developing our soul we initially cultivate a personality in response to people and experiences. It helps us navigate through situations, form relationships and become successful. We also become layered with rules of society, and assumptions and attitudes acquired from our many and varied life experiences.. *Our ego-guided personality is our unique identity in the world—our consistent pattern of presence; our Reliable Self.* While important socially, it is no substitute for character, which is the foundation of a person's life.

The soul is a complex three-fold entity: the lowest soul being the sentient (sensuous) soul of instincts, desires and passions. This force strongly guides and influences our behavior during adolescence and early adulthood. The middle principle is the intellectual or rational soul; the logic and reasoning force that becomes most influential in our actions and behaviors in middle-late adulthood.

The highest member of the soul is beginning conscious awareness itself. Thoughts and emotions are being touched by our inner spirit and intuition is born. As it matures during the second half of life we build an inner spiritual world and moral base for serving humanity. Until we are deeply matured, our human Ego, the bearer of personality and self-consciousness, plays these three soul-members like a musical instrument in an orchestra. In any given situation it will take its 'cues' from sensations, thoughts, or higher knowing to create a response. It is the combined reaction of these three 'souls' that creates harmony or disharmony in our life.

We move from the prescriptive first half of life to the second, where we work into finer development of our inner and outer nature by maturing our soul. The process begins by learning to control our emotions. A second stage of growth occurs as we learn to manage our thoughts. The final stage of soul development occurs as we make decisions using our own higher knowledge, generated by insights learned from the many and varied life experiences we have had. We shed the hierarchy of rules and demands of outer society as we develop self-mastery and moral autonomy. The more we cultivate our soul, the more our spiritual capacities are developed.

Launching into adulthood—ages 21-28—offers opportunities to work on refinement of the sentient soul (instincts, desires and passions). If we are successful in learning to manage these basic emotions, the next phase—ages 28-35—bring issues and experiences that help us refine our intelligence in a moral and ethical way. Focus shifts to looking for the greater good vs. making self-serving decisions that achieve our goals at others expense. The third, and final stage—age 35-42—moves us into the realm where we begin to recognize and know our own self; the witness observer is born who can help us see with discernment and make decisions wisely.

Soul Mirroring
By Age Phases

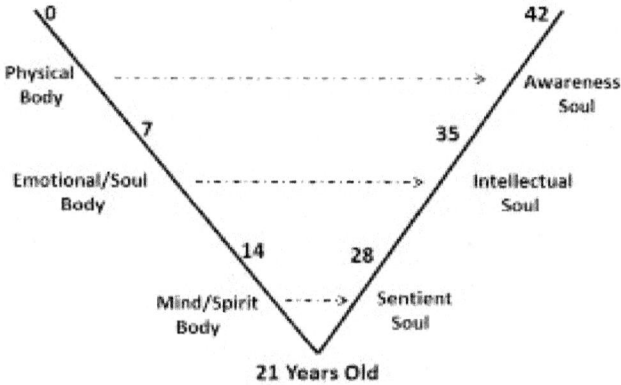

Adapted from Burkhard, 2003, 91

To explore the causes and consequences of your emotional and moral progression during the second stage of your life, utilize the Soul Mirroring Map. Itemize the chronological events of your life, at the appropriate date across from each other as depicted above. This time, identify the event and the feelings that went with them. Arrange them in a mirroring way, starting on top from 0-21, and from below upwards until 42 or whatever age you are now. It is important to observe the elements that appear between age 21-42, as these events are targeted at development of your soul. Identify shifts in awareness—they are usually generated by sorrow, lack of love, physical or emotional pain. When experienced at a certain age they can promote soul growth or, if not worked through, they can generate an extremely introspective and cautious nature as well as a one-sided mind.

Destiny Openings—Taking One's Own Power:

As we move further into our life story, the 'developmental' phases and stages become less prescriptive and more open to individual interpretation. Earlier life forces for growth get used up, offering us, for the first time, the opportunity to manage our life affairs and personal renewal ourselves. *Here is the point of origin of the freedom of man: here responsibility is born.*

In every moment of life we are moving towards our 28th year, or away from it. Only the years between 28-35 offer an unfiltered experience; we experience life and simultaneously understand it. The first Stage of life is a prescribed path without much choice. The later years mirror back events and relationships from earlier times, so they are laced with previous encounters and all the emotions and assumptions we acquired. *The fulcrum for stepping into our own power and destiny begins during that 6th Phase of development*

Destiny Openings
Ages 18, 37 & 56

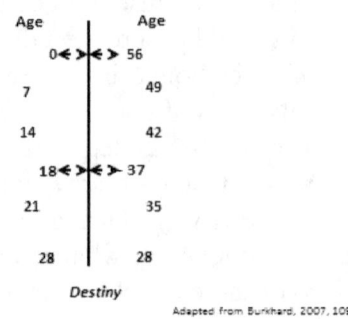

Adapted from Burkhard, 2007, 109

We each come with a predetermined destiny. As the years go by, we get layered with 'baggage', as well as lessons learned. At 18 ½, 37, and again at 56, a 'clearing' occurs. There is an opening event, often powerful and many times uncomfortable, that will put us 'back on track'. Remember that dates and years are approximate; some arrive earlier and others later, but the universal pattern is set.

Using your biographical map, identify the significant life events that address your decision-making regarding career and leadership development, self-identity and a shift in values, and finally on when you focused on the future and the end of your life as well as what you would like to leave behind. Place them into the Destiny Openings matrix.

If you are 55 or older, pay special attention to the <u>final Destiny Opening around age 55 ½</u>. The major question being asked this time is 'How am I to move forward into the future? What do I leave behind'? In this inquiry we can sense our intentions as well as what our real task on earth is. We ponder, 'How have I made a mark in the world'? From this we determine what new tasks we want to undertake, which ones to wrap up, and what could be left behind.

Examine your biography and see if/where a shift towards free choice first occurred. It is often a time of shedding old hierarchical rules and expectations. Note where something new emerged in relation to your taking additional responsibility. If we make this turning point towards our own power prematurely, an early hardening comes about making us obsessive and compulsive. If the fulcrum is delayed too long, it becomes hard for the individual to accept responsibility.

SPIRITUAL DEVELOPMENT-THIRD LIFE CYCLE

Spiritual development optimally occurs between the ages of 42-63; the period of human fulfillment. The fruits of our efforts ripen during this time. Our mature ego opens the door to the cultivation of inner space which is being potentiated by the refocused vital life force. We increasingly become aware of and deepen our connection with the resources inherent within the dark recesses of our higher mind. The single biggest difference in this maturing cycle is that it is not something we can 'learn'. It is something we 'become'.

Personality is replaced with wisdom and authenticity. The core of our character lies within our 'I' individuality; until life is individual it is not moral, it is borrowed or copied. Our thoughts and actions must emerge from the reservoir of our cultivated inner space rather than a rule or law.

Character is our moral compass which encounters and withstands the shock of change and things outward. It comes from a life that directs itself rather than reacting to pressures and expectations from the outside. It is the hallmark of our authentic 'I'—our inner world. Self-mastery is central to the cultivation of spirit and character. The soul's journey is to replace reactions from feeling-based instincts, desires and impulses, to control over them. A maturing soul increasingly directs its will and intentions. Life becomes a disciplined and intelligent journey rather than an emotional roller coaster as we successfully complete this stage of development.

Spiritual development entails maturing of new organs of perception: broader and more effective ways of thinking, feeling and acting. The twelve senses deepen in their sensitivity as intuition expands. Insights and understanding gained from life's lessons are increasingly applied in real time, to whatever comes before us. We put aside rules, logic and thought, as well as deep concern for the past or the future—it is what it is. And we are equipped to deal with whatever comes. Two of the greatest transformational elements for the deepening our spirit include:

o   Perceptual awareness can be dramatically altered by a life-changing tragedy: the contradiction of a disease; a sever accident; death of a parent, child or spouse; a deep betrayal. Such events will turn us bitter or cynical, or will foster the discovery of energies of soul and feelings of love and compassion unknown prior to the event. Tests that challenge our physical and mental abilities deepen or destroy our spirit.

o   Important and often overlooked or undervalued, are the exceptional impression made upon us by a casual acquaintance in earlier life or the quiet influence from those we were associated with for many years. Equally impactful is the sudden appearance of someone we met for a brief moment, who either inspired us deeply or brought great harm upon us. Another opening moment may come from a temptation that overtook us, evil thoughts or imaginings which plagued us, a bad decision that got us into a great deal of trouble. All of these are the outgrowth of germs planted in our minds by persons whom we may not even recall, apart from the harm done.

Mirroring for spiritual development begins at age 31 ½. Each 7-year cycle starts slowly, reaches its peak mid-cycle, and then dwindles towards the end. The issues/opportunities of an earlier stage are repeated again as indicated by the connecting lines. This time you may wish to map your biographical moments into the 9 Cycles of Development template. Instead of selecting events you may choose relationships since our growth spiritually comes most often from deep connections with others.

9 Cycles of Conscious Development
Spiritual Development Begins at 31 ½

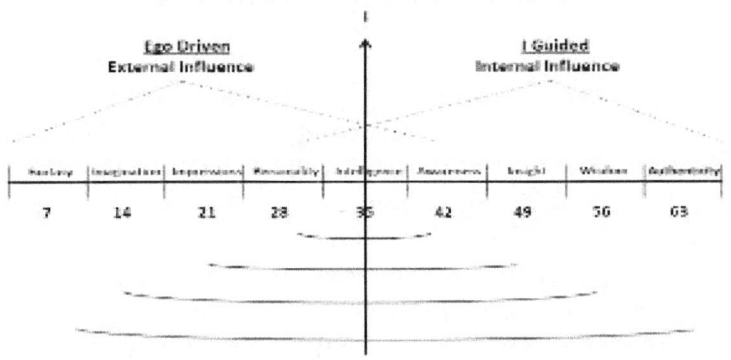

Adapted from Burkhard, 2007, 134

Identify the important people in your life at each stage of development. Then note the people you are in relation to at the present moment., recognizing ones you are close to, and ones are more distant. In this way you will be able to identify if the connection is physical, spiritual or soulful in nature. You can discern which have died (physically or meaning-wise), which are simply being maintained out of a sense of duty, and which have a vital energy within them. Mapping relationships helps us see what is still life-giving, and what should be trimmed and released from our life. You may return to old relationships that still hold an energetic charge, positive or negative, and bring them into harmony and balance. It is not necessary to do this physically, but important that you do so emotionally as forgiveness (of self and/or the other) is essential to the healing of memories

.

IINTEGRATION—THE FORTH LIFE CLCLE

From the age of 63 onwards, we start to free ourselves from the web of destiny. A sense of rebirth sweeps through us as we find the earlier stages running together, with little influence on our reality. Attention turns increasingly towards social and charitable endeavors. The possibility of deep spiritual development is high, and we have many moments to practice when surrounded with older persons who have not taken the path of personal development at mid-life. We select places that offer beauty, rest, education and affirmation, staying away from elders who simply complain or grumble about their health or the state of the world.

As we map the first half of our life against the second half, patterns and issues leap off the page that hold significance for us. By identifying what we learned, and how it was applied to future issues/challenges, we increasingly appreciate the courage and creativity, the, wisdom and intelligence we used in crafting and navigating our life. As we note the mistakes made and intentional hurtful expressions we put into the world, we have a deeper self-compassion, recognizing the challenges inherent in human nature. This translates into a sense of greater acceptance and extended forgiveness to others as we realize we all share together in the complexity of the human condition.

To explore the issues that influenced your spiritual awakening that require integration, place critical life events into the Life Integration matrix. Unlike normal developomental moments (starting high school, etc.) these are the events that are emotionally laden or those of o transitional nature where an event or decision changed the direction ofy our life completely.

Life Integration
By Age Phases

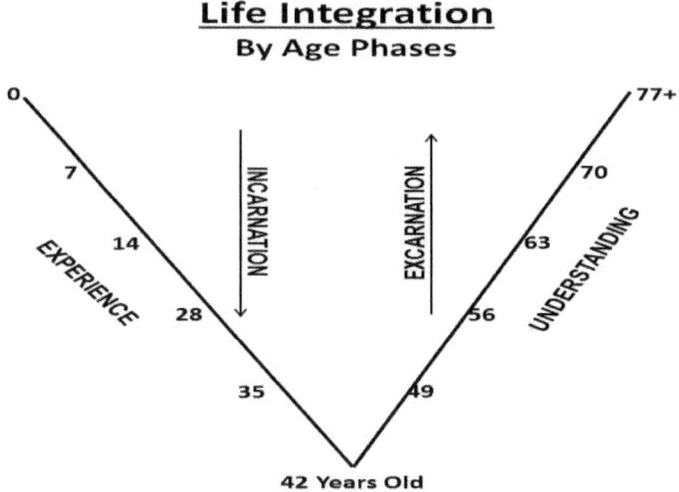

Looking back on our life story from this vantage point, we can recognize the reappearance of certain experiences, behaviors or patterns that await our acceptance and integration. Once we can understand and take them for what they are—we are freed from repeating them again.

At times you will see a significant event on the experience side mirrored across in a similar experience on the understanding side. We ponder questions such as: 'What might I have done better? What made that success so powerful? Where did the friction arise that is causing difficulties in our inter-personal relationship? Is there still time to rectify a troubling issue or pattern in this lifetime'? If we throw light on our own life story, we pass through death less burdened. We experience—death by completion.

A Living Example of Authentic Connection

Here is an entry from a journal made by an 82 year old woman who was suffering from end-stage cancer. She was living in a hospice unit, confined to her bed. Only the view outside her window was available to her.

Birds singing, rain falling softly on the windowpane—pain.

I tap on the window of my inner world. I slip into deep relaxation and reverie, the dark warm water of my inner world. It is comforting here.

We need to believe in the beauty within. Nurture it. Link it with the beauty and mystery of a larger existence. Serve one with the other. Feed off it and serve it.

A great work grows out of the unspoken, the half-understood, the subconscious. There is a wisdom inside each of us that cannot be put into words but it can, with practice, be accessed to guide and shape our lives and our work. It has elements of the holy about it.

To offer beauty and love as you go through life, you need to live in connection with your inner world. This is all I have left. It is more than enough. It is abundance. I am fulfilled."

Part III

My Way: Mindful Life Choices
What do you think you are doing?

*Health is not
the equivalent to happiness or
success. It is foremost a matter of
being wholly one with whatever
circumstances we find ourselves in.
Even death is a healthy event if
we fully embrace the fact of our
dying. The issue is awareness of
living in the present. Whatever our
present existence consists of, if we
re at one with it we are healthy.*

Elizabeth Kubler-Ross

Chapter 7

Health & Illness:
Choosing Health

> A wise person should consider that health is
> the greatest of human blessings, and learn how
> by his own thought to derive benefit from his
> illnesses.
> Hippocrates

Where were you living when you were age 12? Who was taking care of you at that time? What happened to you when you became ill? Were you pampered and supported, or shamed and told to 'keep going!'? We each carry a definition of health, and multiple experiences of it in our lives. These personal beliefs and life experiences color every thought and conversation we have about this important aspect of our life experience—our health and wellbeing.

Individuals who view health as the absence of disease spend their life on trying to 'combat' illness with antibiotics, surgery and other treatments targeting the physical body. Others view health as mind/body/spirit balance, and spend time and effort on the physical, emotional and spiritual dimensions of their life to enhance well-being. A smaller groups takes a broader view of health as 'an 'expansion of awareness'.

Dr. Margaret Newman took care of her aging and dying mother. She discovered that the more restricted and bedridden her mother became, the 'healthier' she got. Her attitude of appreciation and understand kept enlarging as she lost her physical abilities, one by one. At her death she was 'whole' in her comprehension of life in all its many dimensions and the gifts of understanding it had bestowed upon her. Filled with wisdom and gratitude, she experienced a peaceful death. How you define 'health' determines what you will do to acquire and/or maintain it.

A MODEL OF HUMAN HEALTH

Contemporary definitions of health refer to wholeness: the ability to live in harmony with your surroundings yet separately; the ability to set yourself apart independently without isolating yourself or rejecting others; the ability to open yourself up in authentic relationships without becoming dissolved.

The World Health Organization defines health as bodily, spiritual and social well-being. It is not a fixed state, but dynamic and always changing. Our body is in a constant state of shifting to obtain harmony within its many parts and functions. Modern Western Medicine explores illness by following factors which cause illness. Eastern Medicine treats illness by supporting internal forces that maintain or restore health.

Complete Health combines the best of all worlds and gives you tools and resources to treat each and every aspect of your fourfold self. Beyond the absence of disease, it is a flourishing sense of well-being; sound in body, mind and spirit. A healthy population is a resilient population that can grow an economy and help create the kind of society that helps people thrive.

Four Elements of Wholeness:

Four principles are at work in every human being. All elements of being human are contained in these four principles: a- the material (physical) body; b- the vital (biological) life processes; c- the soul (mental/emotional) elements; and d- the individual mind (self/'I') awareness. These four elements are in constant interaction in every person. The specific interaction pattern for each of us gives rise to the uniqueness and character of our individual nature.

4 Body Model: Body, Vitality, Mind & Spirit
Elements of Human Wholeness

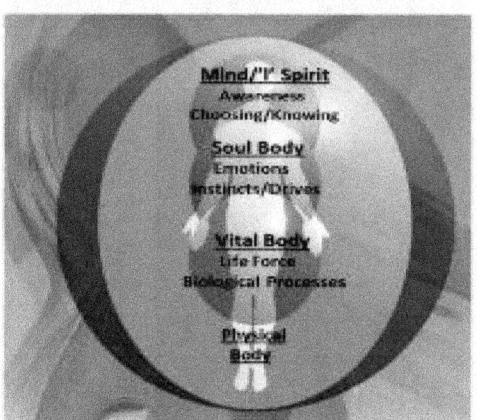

The physical (material) body: All parts of the physical body can be weighed, counted or measured. As part of the mineral world, it is subject to natural laws of nature. The physical body is the outer, visible form of the human being with a *Mechanical Intelligence*: it inherently functions in accordance with laws of physics and gravity. We do not have to think about how our arm will bend or how to shift weight to maintain our balance in activities of daily living—mechanical wisdom provides this adjusting function.

The life vitality (biological) body: The flow of life energy can be found in a plant, animal or human. It brings about life through seven rhythmic processes which are closely interrelated in a state of delicate balance. While it is not visible to the eye, vitality is recognized by the state of energy and health felt within the body. During the first half of life this energy is focused on development and maintenance of the physical body. After mid-life the energy increasingly shifts to developmental tasks of the soul. An inner space is established, along with a second set of 'senses' that cultivate wisdom during the second half of life.

Throughout life energy pulsates through the whole body and it is through the rhythms of this 'life vitality' that we maintain our own biological state. These 7 life processes include:

o   Life coming to us—our primary relationships with the outer world:
    Breathing – taking in air; the breath of life. Through breath we connect and disconnect with the world in a rhythmic manner. Oxygen is a critical fuel for bodily chemical interactions. During the second half of life this also includes our power of observation—how we 'take in' the larger world.

    Warming – adjusting temperature for optimal interaction. The right warmth enables bodily functions to interrelate optimally. During the second half of life this also refers to warmth in physical and emotional relating; the enthusiasm to draw towards or turn away from something or someone in our lives.

    Nourishing – taking in food; ingesting nourishment provides energy and strength. During the second half of life this increasingly refers to how we digest or assimilate life lessons, the struggle between the old and the new and our own intentions.

o   Life within us:
    Secreting – the first internal process is most critical—its primary function is to secrete what it does not need. It is

114

the principle of distinguishing between what is essential and what is non-essential. In the second half of life it is the principle of simplification of one's life.

Maintaining – functioning in a way that preserves form and function of the body for ongoing life. Rest and sleep allow for maintenance and repair of the body. In the second half of life maintenance is enhanced by increasingly experiencing a sense of peace and trust, facilitating balanced wholeness in our daily life.

Growing – Life force requires not only simply maintenance, but also the impulse for growth. In the first half of life vital energy focuses on development of the physical body. After mid-life growth forces turn to the soul for the integration of life lessons to obtain wisdom.

Reproducing – When the six vital functions are balanced, one has the ability to bring about a new form which is a replication of the old; body regeneration. After midlife reproduction is experienced in becoming more authentic by creating our own unique interpretation of and response to life.

The life processes are silent and unseen; but their presence (or absence) is always recognized. They flow through our body guided by *Biological Intelligence,* following the laws of the natural and biological sciences. We do not have to tell ourselves to breathe faster when we run and need more oxygen, chemical monitors in our body will adjust rate of breath and rate of movement to maintain vital balance.

The soul (mental/emotional) body: Our soul concerns itself with our instincts, drives and an inner sense of the world around us. Our feelings, which are obvious to us, cannot be observed by others, but our behavior can. We feel pain when our body is hurt, and we also feel an inner pain when our feelings are hurt. In the soul all life sensations and movements have their home.

Impressions from the outer world awaken our thoughts and stir our feelings – sight, hearing, smell, taste, touch, temperature, and balance. They are experienced and interpreted in our soul. *Emotional Intelligence* guides our response to each life encounter with a sense of attraction or repulsion. This series of sense activity happens on different levels:

o   In the physical body your brain will recognize and register feelings and perceptions sensed in/by the body.

o   In the emotional soul those perceptions are felt and categorized as either a sense of 'like' or 'dislike'.

o   In the 'I' (spirit) your mind –*Spiritual Intelligence* or higher authority—clarifies those feelings, lifts them into your conscious awareness, and makes a choice regarding whether to move forward or hold back.   Your intentions determine the direction and outcomes desired.

In the first twenty one years of life this process is automatic. However, the older we become the more we settle into habitual and patterned ways of seeing and acting. To move from reacting out of old patterns, a conscious commitment to continuous learning and further development must be made. If we get into the practice on reviewing each situation with fresh eyes, we will have a lifetime of learning. If we react unconsciously, we will have one year of life repeated over and over again. Maturing across the lifespan requires a commitment to your own growth—consciously— moment by moment each day.

The individual (self-conscious mind) 'I' body: Each of us lives in the here-and-now, taking on responsibility for our life within our culture. As independent personalities we are able to make our own decisions. 'I' can make a choice that can satisfy or thrill me, go against my natural inclinations, or even my feelings. Each of us is an 'I', living in a unique world of our own, the center point of our own individual life and existence. Along with making choices, this self-aware part of our being can innovate and create something new. Our unique thoughts and actions form our specific contribution to the world.

From birth to death, life is maintained and physical development occurs as long as Mechanical and Biological Intelligence guide the interaction between material and vital life processes. When we add the unseen components of Emotional and Spiritual Intelligence, we also transform our opinions and beliefs with insights gained from our lived experience. This expands our understanding and our options, moving us towards higher, more inclusive order—*we acquire freedom and wisdom.* (NOTE: using the word spiritual does not imply health based on beliefs, or religious factors. It refers to the self-conscious life-force that runs through us all—organizing our body elements, monitoring our feelings and enlightening our awareness.)

COMPLETE HEALTH

Complete Health combines the best of all worlds and gives you tools and resources to treat each every aspect of your fourfold self.

Bodily well-being: A healthy body has the ability to react sensibly and adequately to the continuously changing conditions and influences to which you as a human being are exposed. *Adaptation* occurs both within the body, and between the body and its environment when there is a healthy exchange or action between them. From this point of view, people with a disability or chronic condition can, through the use of assistive devices and prosthetics, cope with their situation in such a way that they live a healthy life. They live with the disease rather than as the disease.

Social well-being: A healthy emotional/soul life is necessary for a sense of social well-being. *Coherence* is 'the feeling of being at one with all there is'. People in coherence feel themselves appreciated by and at home in society. This is especially meaningful during the extreme situations of great happiness and extreme sorrow. Sharing in crisis strengthens the vital life force. Knowing someone is there who understands gives courage to endure the worst situations, even if the other person is not close by physically. It is equally important to give support to others, for this also strengthens the health of one's soul. It is a basic human need to be of social significance to others.

Spiritual well-being: A strong spirit, or essential self, has the ability to be *resilient.* From this stance one has the strength to withstand attacks of negative, destructive and hostile influences that can cause depression and illness. Special attention should be paid to personal sorrow. We often experience powerlessness when confronted by violence, brutality or catastrophes of magnitude, especially when we are unable to grasp their meaning or do anything about them. Resilience fosters strength that keeps us from breaking down. Instead. we develop trust in the meaningful evolution of humanity while discovering the sense of purpose in our own life. People who are spiritually healthy will be able to see their destiny, whatever it is, in a wider context; they can accept and deal with things because they take the position which gives them confidence to open up their perspective for their future.

DISTURBANCES IN HEALTH

Body processes are always at work, giving us a sense of vitality and well-being. Symptoms of illness, before they become pathological, are healthy capacities (i.e., secretions, warmth, sensitivity, etc.). They are considered illness only when they occur at the wrong place, at the wrong time and with the wrong intensity. If they become too strong or weak, an illness has begun. The further it progresses, the harder it is to reverse the process.

Bodily Illness:

Whether the imbalance is expressed as a defense reaction, excessive or inadequate functioning, insufficiency, cramps, paralysis, tumors or other bodily symptoms, the body is seeking a healthy balanced middle position as it struggles between the two opposing forces of strength and disintegration.

' Anthroposophic Medicine' refers to the imbalances which appear as symptoms of illness, as 'cold' or 'warm' illnesses. Cold illnesses comprise all those that tend towards denseness or blockages that lead to hardening, stones, cramps and degenerative disease. In warm illnesses, on the other hand, the loosening processes are too strong. Such illnesses tend towards the direction of fever, hypersecretion, swelling and inflammation.

Balancing Life Processes

Too Hot- Too Cold

Too Much – Too Little

Too Firm – Too Slack

Too Hard – Too Soft

Too Tense – Too Flaccid

Too Dry – Too Wet

Adapted from Camps, 2006, p.61

Generally speaking, illnesses in the first half of life tend to be more inflammatory in nature, while degenerative conditions increasingly occur in older age. Because illnesses often have biographical significance, one must look at similar illnesses in a different way at various phases of life development: each case is unique to the individual.

Soul-Related Illnesses: This category of illnesses occurs when an inner sense of coherence is lost. It is the nature of your soul to live in polarities as there are an infinite number of ways to express the ecstasy of joy and doldrums of despair. We live in a constant state of exchange between our inner and outer world. In our social life we swing between the need to be with others and the need to have solitude and alone time. A well-balance person can find the middle between those extremes; i.e., being as happy on their own as being sociable in the company of others.

Extreme emotional swings require psychiatric intervention, but for most people, shifting moods are a normal part of life. We are constantly in a state of psychological flow, changing situations foster corresponding emotional feelings. Soul illnesses share many qualities of physical illness: the process of hardening takes on the qualities of anxieties, depressions, compulsions and self-destructive tendencies. The process of loosening manifests as a state of delusion, hallucination and loss of limits. As with physical illness, the root cause of an emotional or mental illness is to be identified and treated. Because the language of the soul is symbols and sounds, art and music therapy are excellent tools for therapeutic intervention.

Spiritual Illnesses: A basic anthroposphic principle is that spirit itself cannot become ill. What can occur, however, is impairment of a healthy spirit. Illness in the body or soul hinders the sound spirit from finding healthy expression in our life. This is experienced as a loss of meaning for existence. Emotions and environmental factors play a central role in an illness event. The resilient human spirit had unlimited potential to adapt, adjust, or course-correct an injured body or mind/thought pattern in a 'healing experience'. Or, in death the spirit leaves the body without dying itself.

ILLNESS AND DESTINY

The human life journey includes both health and illness. Illnesses are often a part of the life story—signaling that something must change. The cause for illness can often be found in the past; one's life style, nutritional or environmental pattern may have led to the disturbance, deficiency or damage. The injured organism demands appropriate compensation and a change in life circumstances.

A physical illness can become a developmental opportunity for the person, especially if it is properly cared for and not suppressed. It can become a 'shortened biography'—if the illness had not occurred it would take longer for that same person to mature. The question of what causes illness remains open to the individual who is affected. If the past does not hold clues, attention must shift to the future. When one looks (with the help of a healthy spirit) for a wider context, we see that if others also have had a similar challenge—it is a developmental phase task. Or, we note that no one else has had a similar situation and recognize the illness as a challenge of destiny. In such a circumstance it is necessary to question the meaning of the illness: "What does this illness mean for me? Can I learn from it? Where does it come from? Where will it lead"?

To achieve and maintain the delicate balance of health is a dynamic and ongoing process. When illness strikes we come to recognize our own limits in coping with stress and other factors that threaten our health. We often learn new coping mechanisms and faculties that may be an enrichment to our life, strengthening our self-healing capacity.

While specific care in and of itself cannot heal, it does create conditions for our body to heal itself. On a bodily level, the right kind of care will support our life forces. On the level of soul, it can bring about helpful personal encounters which will strengthen the balance of soul emotions and feeling of coherence. On the spiritual level, care helps individuals recognize their uniqueness and helps them find a path of life that is in harmony with what their destiny wants.

A Living Example of Health as Your Teacher

Jeff Casebolt is an Outward Bound Instructor—and a cancer patient. Here are his thoughts about living with a life-threatening illness.

Sometimes we have to travel to the edge of ourselves to find our center.
                                    - Buck Ghost Horse, Lakota Medicine Man

"I've always been attracted to the edge in life. Boxing, hitchhiking north in my teens to fight forest fires with Dogrib Indians. Whitewater kayaking. Out on the edge, unpredictable things happen. New combinations, new understandings, emerge. Even cancer, in its own way, was a journey along the edge. I had to be alone. I had to confront myself and how I was living. I had to change how I lived to survive. Before it was all gone. I won't say I enjoyed cancer because I definitely didn't, but there was an exciting aspect to it.

Challenging doctors and their self-satisfied approach to medicine was fun, for instance. "So, doctor, you seem pretty certain about what I should do next. Tell me, what percentage of patients survive with what I've got following your advice?" They had an extensive knowledge of the problem. When it came to the solution, their confidence, to the extent they had any, was not comforting. I was on my own.

You have to consult with your heart. That doesn't wash over very well in a society that needs empirical evidence for everything. "What are your rational reasons for doing this trip? For making this choice?" A lot of the most important decisions we make aren't rational. I'm coming to appreciate that more and more. Sometimes, when you get to higher levels or deeper levels, things become less and less certain. You run out of facts and figures and you have to turn inward and really consult your sense about what is right and true for you. This trip will serve me all my life in terms of allowing me to be more of an individual. Freer from social rules about what is right, what I should do. Honor and live my truth.

That two and a half years changed me. It's so challenging internally to travel day after day by yourself. And have to face yourself day after day. To have to stew in your own psyche and your own loneliness. You are forced to look at yourself. You are forced to look, look inward. Who am I? What's here? ... It's something that I will carry with me for the rest of my life. A journey like that is both external and internal. I experienced the most incredible range of emotional highs and lows. I confronted the most incredible existential loneliness. The trip expanded me on every level. My desire for spiritual depth and awareness was one result. I encountered amazing people — encountered highs and lows within myself — that I could not have otherwise accessed. The trip was a glacier that gouged internally. The marks are indelibly inscribed in my soul.

Life is a mystery. Everything — where we came from, where we are going, the nature of life, the spark (what created it?) — the ends of the universe — all the big questions are mysterious. You encounter the mystery on adventures. You embrace life on adventures. And you get beat up. But hopefully not beaten down.

If you really know what things you want out of life, it's amazing how opportunities will come to enable you to carry them out. On your death bed, will you wish you had taken more risks or fewer? Which would have offered a richer experience of existence? Which would have best honored that precious gift—your life? Live on the edge!

Chapter 8

Successful Aging:
The Wisdom Phase

> The young person knows the
> rules, but the wise elder knows the
> exceptions. The best way to know
> the future is to invent it.
> Oliver Wendell Holmes

L ike the childhood and adult phases of life, old age is a life
  stage in which a developmental process is still taking
  place. Though our bodily forces decrease and
surroundings get more confined, it is in no way to be viewed
as a decline. It is rather a time when various aspects of being
human undergo characteristic changes. Whereas in the first
half of life the vital life force is focused primarily on the
physical body, the second half of life is dedicated to the
development of soul and spirit utilizing those forces now
freed from the body. It is the decline of the physical body
that makes spiritual growth possible.

A MODEL FOR AGING

When does aging begin? With the first breath of life. Our
life is a cycle, moving from incarnation at birth to excarnation
at death.

The Cycle of Life
By Age Phases

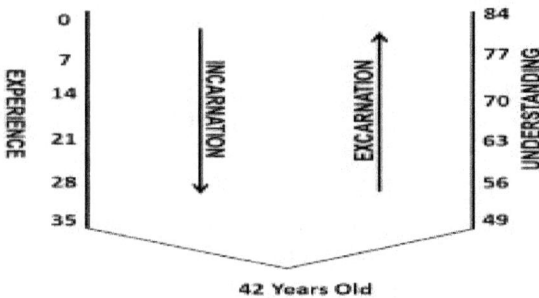

42 Years Old

Adapted from Burkhard, 1997 p.168

A person who is at the peak of social effectiveness and responsibility in the outer world takes a decisive turn inward at mid-life. The human life span gives us the first half of life in which to generate many experiences, while in the second half of life we learn to understand life to in general, and your own life in particular, to help deepen your soul and spirit in a manner that leads to wisdom and a death of completion.

At mid-life we are given a choice; "*to begin actively developing the 'higher soul/spirit bodies' and become more fully human, or to remain in the patterns and cycles of the first half of life and rigidify into a 'mummy' through their life routine* (Rudolph Steiner). Successful aging requires purposeful self-development after age 42.

AGING OF THE FOUR BODIES

Aging has a specific set of tasks and assignments to be accomplished during the final stage of life. No phase is exempt from continued growth and development.

The Physical Body in Old Age: At biological mid-life (age 35-42) the physical body becomes more subject to aging. It is increasingly difficult for the life forces to regenerate the body. The body becomes denser and drier, loses flexibility, becoming more fragile. Vital functions are diminishing as blood pressure rises, metabolism is less able to cope with food intake, vessels become harder and hearing, eyesight and the growth of hair diminishes. The signs and symptoms of aging become increasingly visible in our face, our skin and our gate.

The Vital Body in Old Age: With respect to the life forces in the physical body multiple signs of aging appear in functioning. The reproductive faculty in women comes to an end. Breathing becomes shallower and less body warmth is produced. Body maintenance becomes slower (i.e., healing of wounds). Physical changes appear (i.e., age-related patches on the skin) and growths may occur (i.e. tumors). Excretions become slacker leading to dry skin and some allergies.

When these life forces are less tied to the body, they can be freed up for energizing a higher plane. An earlier freeing of the life forces occurred when the child changed teeth in their youth. This energy assisted them for use in learning in school. Because life cycles are continuous and repetitive, this freeing up of the life force is once again put to use in assisting our education in thinking—we are given power for emergence of deeper intelligence gained from our life experiences.

The seven life processes are now capable of taking on a more subtle capacity, fostering 'the wisdom of age':

o *Breathing:* Outer impressions and inner beliefs are taken to a deeper level
o *Warming:* A deep and affectionate warm enthusiasm can be developed for the world and the spiritual essence behind it (i.e., philosophy, art, religion)
o *Nourishing:* Thoughts are less superficial, taken to a deeper level and 'digested', resulting in a deeper understanding of the world, life and people in general
o *Secreting:* A new definition emerges as to what is essential and what is not. Every day events are less interesting(fluid thinking), while greater insights arise concerning the 'big questions of life' (crystalline thinking)

126

- o *Maintaining:* Greater connections are perceived, and with age we gain a wider vista for observation and understanding
- o *Growing:* The aging person develops a rich inner life, a sanctuary for the soul that is filled with beauty, truth and peace
- o *Reproducing:* Due to a greater overview, life-experience and understanding of how things are connected and how they work, the aging person can achieve mature thoughts, understanding and creations that are of lasting value

In the second half of life, if these forces turn mainly to the physical and material body and are not used for deeper spiritual development, disturbances in the body can occur.

Emotional/Soul Body in old age: Feelings of sadness are normal as they arise in the soul at the loss of beauty and a former way of life. Loss is a doorway into compassion for oneself, for humanity and the world. Bitterness can also be felt at the loss of bodily pleasures, kindling a desire to compensate by other means that foster intensity of experience (i.e., extravagances, misuse of medicines, flashy jewelry, lavish new home or car, sexual encounters, etc.). Or, specialists may be sought that will minimize the effects of aging, or provide drugs which will free the person from age-related miseries.

Whether we gracefully accept, or totally reject the process of aging, deep down we know that its progression cannot be halted through outer manipulation. The initial dissatisfaction felt as aging becomes increasingly seen and felt can evoke a redefinition of one's life. While not stressing a fragile body too much, contemplative walks, age appropriate dance and gym, creative pass times, music and artistic adventures bring movement to the soul through the rhythms of tension and relaxation. Friends, family, fellowship and festivals offer a chance for connection and celebration. New capacities will be developed that compensate for outer loss by gains in inner richness.

'Taking Leave' is an important, and increasingly frequent, experience in the aging process. Attending memorial gatherings for those who have died helps the soul experience both the joy of memories and dignified sorrow regarding loss. This ritual helps aging folks gradually loosen their attachment to earthly things and appreciate that it is the immortal aspects of self—soul and spirit—that carry and support them to the end. Making use of all available strengths while accepting one's limits, allows our soul to swing between rest and activity, arriving at peaceful composure.

The individual 'I' Spirit in old age: The world of the elderly becomes increasingly smaller. Fewer people remain who have lived through the same part of history as they have. Those remaining have less mobility, reducing the number of shared gatherings. Friends and relatives increasingly step into the background as they get busy with their own lives, or they die. Hardly anyone around knows them as they once were. The new generation has other experiences and outlooks on life. New developments in politics and technology, coupled with the emergence of a different value system, are not easily understood by the aging person. Isolation can become an issue at this time.

The loneliness of aging comes from this increasing disconnect with the outer world. Self-confidence must now come from within; strength and support cannot come from a world that is not understood. Inner values of religion and philosophy gain significance; ties with the outer world are released. Trust is increasingly placed in activities of the inner world; new experiences emerge on the journey into this unknown and unfamiliar land. Unique and unpredictable landscapes, paths and insights are of a deeper nature. The kind of progress made is much determined by one's own life story—the attention and care given to purposeful aging across the life span. Biography is a living thing.

The strength of the 'I' determines how much our authentic self will take the lead, how lively the journey will be, and how many experiences will be created or encountered.

Physical and social surroundings can either be a help or a hindrance. The status that is bestowed upon one human being by others influences their personhood. Does contemporary society honor or ignore aged persons? Is the family unit intact or ruptured? The nature of our interaction with the environment and the people in our life will strongly influence whether the spiritual aging process will be experienced as maturation or deterioration.

Illness in old age:

Age related illness can be due to organ deterioration. However, in modern society, with so much toxicity in the environment, including the food we eat, water we drink and air we breathe, our body organs responsible for detoxification (liver, lungs and kidneys) are working overtime. Injury to these vital organs is often the precursor to chronic conditions such as diabetes, lung disease and cancer.

Chronicity and suffering are on the rise world-wide. With the methods and technologies of modern medicine we have increased life span without increasing wellness and health. A question that is increasingly being asked is how do we value the length of life? In view of the increasing number of senior citizens globally, the issue arises whether old age is a burden to society or a blessing. Its hidden meaning may provide humanity with an opportunity to develop capacities which run counter to much of the social coldness, destructiveness and violence of contemporary society.

BECOMING AN ELDER

Successful aging will bring us back to joy! The joy of young children and old adults is similar—with one profound difference. Children are happy because of what they *do not know*, while seniors are happy because of what they *do know*. They have lived long enough to know that everything will eventually work out, irrespective of how it looks at a given moment in time. They also have come to realize a great secret: love is all that matters. Things and power come and go, but meaningful relationships with people, nature, and a Higher Spirit, are the essentials for life—and they are available to everyone.

Markers of the Elder: Several specific qualities emerge in the life of a senior citizen who has reached the maturity of 'elder-hood'. An inner shift occurs that is recognized by the person, and also noted by others with whom they interact. Markers of a wise elder include:

o   *Effortlessness:* Suddenly wisdom matters more than the drama in a situation. There is no felt pressure to fix, intervene or judge. One can associate with another's pain and the need to heal it, but is not drawn into the drama. Engaged, but not attached personally, rather than a swift emotional reaction, deep thought, clarity and a sense of detachment arises regarding the situation at hand. Remaining engaged with an open heart and mind, while absent a strong ego connection, helps bring healing to all in the situation.

o   *Instant Response:* The repercussion of our thoughts and actions occurs almost immediately. Previously we could live in denial (what I just said or did was not harmful to anyone, nor will it affect me). But now we cannot manipulate the truth of what we think, do or say. Negative consequences will show up in insomnia, physical symptoms, or a clear recognition of the situation and our role in it. This clarity and discomfort help us figure out how to fix what is misaligned, and as we learn from the lesson we determine how to stop the thought or behavior from going forward. We become fully accountable for our total self.

Everything done in life has to be processed in old age. This gives us a refined ability to steer our life till the very end. The key to successful aging—without undue disappointments or regrets—is to bring balance into our life review.

Balanced life review: In the beginning of the process there is an inherent tendency to remember only the bad things done to us by others, and the good things we have done. But honest deeper introspection will identify the multiple ways we co-opted the outcome of a difficult situation, and ways in which we deliberately hurt or offended others.

At some point we become filled with awareness accompanied by shame. While it is a natural step in the process, it is dangerous to get stuck there. Making mistakes is built into the human condition; it is the primary vehicle for a thinking and creative mind to learn. Making amends for wrongs done is a preferred way to deal with this clarity of awareness. When that is not possible, an equally effective way of healing the wounds is to *learn the lesson.* Any mistake, no matter how destructive, can be converted to some good effect if we accept responsibility for it and in deep reflection, create understanding and meaning from the situation. In that way, the merit of the event will be recognized and internalized in personal and spiritual growth; it has been redeemed.

Acknowledging mistakes must be balanced with an honest celebration for the good things we have done in our life. We must be as accountable for our successes as our failures. You are then less susceptible to the judgment of others, and you will be less judging as well. Take pride in your work, your life, the path you have walked. Not in a boastful and egocentric way, but with humility stand in the power of knowing that you consistently did your best.

Gracefully become fully who you are, acknowledging and accepting both the negative and positive aspects of your human nature. Taking full accountability for yourself is the key to peaceful aging.

Sharing the wisdom gained: As young adults search for truth, they often experience noble anger at the current state of the world. If supported and encouraged to maintain an honest exchange with life, it turns into goodness and loving kindness with age. A primary responsibility of an elder is to be a guardian of the inquiring young minds waking up to the realities of life.

Central to this exchange of wisdom is honesty. It is important to share past life experiences and lessons learned. This must include the things that we, individually and collectively as a generational cohort, did in the situation under consideration. Telling what was done right as well as what we did wrong gives both insight and permission to make mistakes and learn from them.

The one thing younger people are seeking from seniors is authenticity. They do not want someone to 'be young' like they are. Adults who try to remain 'youthful' are rejected because the younger generation can find that quality within their own cohort. An elder who is real, authentic, creative, interesting and honest models a way of being that they want to evolve into. Well- grounded elders are a central force in fostering hope and inspiration in the young.

There is a pressing need to develop new models of health and aging. Only when we recognize that every stage— including the final one—is a container for experiencing change which fosters growth and insight, can we move forward with openness and resolve. Any age can be the best age if we respect it for what it is, and align with it in a way that fosters further understanding, wisdom and peace.

A Living Example of Successful Aging:

Henry James is a celebrated author who composed many notable books and novels in his life, not each one a success. Consider how he dealt with the many setbacks and rejections throughout his career.

"The consolation, the dignity, the joys of life that flow from discouragements and lapses, depressions and darknesses, come to one only

*as one stands outside of themselves -- I mean outside the luminous
paradise of my work. Disconnected and silent, I see the beauty and joy
of emptiness—my soul expands. As soon as I re-enter my work ,
refreshed-- cross the loved threshold -- stand in the high chamber, and the
gardens divine -- the whole realm widens out again before me and around
me -- the air of life fills my lungs -- the light of achievement flushes over
all the place, and I believe! I see! I do!*
—Henry James

James, one of the great writers of the late 1800s and early
1900s, wrote those words at a low point in his career. He was
struggling financially. He had just finished a play which he
hoped would restore his financial situation. It failed; the
audience threw vegetables onto the stage at the opening. The
next morning, James wrote in his journal:

"Produce; produce again; produce better than ever and all will be well."

And he did produce. He wrote over 20 novels, dozens of
short stories and plays, books of travel, biography and
autobiography.

One of the things that made him great, in addition to his
devotion to his craft, was that he didn't give up, didn't stop
writing when his work met with derision. He worked
through the failures and gained strength in the process. An
artist (person) works with imperfection; if the starting point is
perfection, there's nowhere to go, nothing to create. And as
human beings, we work with our own imperfection. Someone
who has finished searching, has all the answers, has nothing
to learn, cannot create. Creating any piece of art or a
meaningful life is a search into realms where truth can be
sensed but not seen. The big truths, the truths that are the
territory of art (and life), are contradictory.

James understood that beauty includes freedom from the
perfect. Beauty encompasses the infinite, and the infinite by
necessity encompasses freedom. Items made by machines
can be perfect. Items made by hand, including art, cannot be

both perfect and have a soul. To give energy, to enlarge one's concept of the potentials of life, a work of art (one's life) must contain mistakes. Mistakes reflect where the artist was, what the artist's state of mind was, at the moment of execution. It is the things left out, deliberately or unintentionally, the things hidden, the things not fully executed or complete, that suggest, point to, life beyond the poem (the painting, the moment, the day).

Chapter 9

Death & Dying:
Death by Completion

> There is no real
> ending. It is just the
> place where you stop the
> story.
> Frank Herbert

The human being was not designed for immortality. We enter into our body with a finite number of years existence programmed into it. Aging is the process designed to expose us to multiple experiences from differing vantage points so that we can continue to learn and transform, evolving always towards our most full and authentic self. All of life is progression towards wholeness.

Anthroposophy regards the human as a reincarnating being. The 'I' spirit, the individual core of a human being, comes to earth to have experiences and take responsibility for them. It enters upon your first breath, and leaves with the last exhalation. With death life is not finished, it takes on a new form of existence that begins as the 'I' processes and evaluates the experiences of the life completed and integrates them into itself. Each successive lifetime gives us the ability to practice and strengthen capacities and insights gained from the last incarnation. The design of repeated lives on earth is

135

that each of us, step by step, can perfect ourselves until we have reached the next stage of development.

This view of multiple lives helps us understand that there is not just one single opportunity. If we have failed in our efforts we will have multiple other opportunities to try again to achieve our goals. Each significant event, favorable or difficult, is an important life experience that helps us gain new forces, capabilities and understandings. The consequences of a chain of subtle causes, they serve as a preparation to acquire new skills and knowledge that will assist us in the next set of tasks which may arise in later incarnations.

A MODEL FOR DEATH & REINCARNATION

Our physical body contains and supports the other three aspects of being human. It belongs to the earth, carried by our mother from conception to birth. Over a period of time, step by step, the vital body, emotional soul and 'I' spirit also incarnate. At middle life, Cycle 2, they are closely linked together and all is closely connected to the earth. Towards the end of the second cycle the other bodies gradually begin to loosen from the physical body and the path towards excarnation is begun.

As the loosening progresses, the life processes begin to exert less influence over the physical body and it begins to dry up. The vital life energy increasingly is used to enhance soul and 'I' development; deeper consciousness is born. The loss of vitality physically causes our human body to lose its former shape. We begin to notice wrinkles, loss of energy, diminished muscle tone, and a host of other symptoms of aging. Those structuring forces are now available for the life of your soul. While your body is aging, you are given a freer unfolding of thinking and emotional maturity. Increasingly your 'I' assumes the role of holding together and ordering your thinking and soul-life to develop it further. This explains our mid-life crisis shift.

Dying is that final stage in life where your 'I', emotional-soul body and life processes clearly separate from the physical body. The moment of death marks the completion of this separation as your higher human parts 'cross the threshold'.

Physical body after death: The first body to deteriorate after death is your physical body. As the vital life force leaves the body it becomes inert and returns to earth as dead matter. The other three bodies are still interconnected in the immediate surroundings of the earth but they are free of the body.

Vital life body after death: As your vital life body releases from the physical body immediately upon death it provides your 'I' spirit with an image of what was imprinted on it during the course of your life. There is a recorded memory of every moment in your life, whether you were consciously aware of it or not. People who have had a near-death experience frequently describe this life review as a big panorama with all the images side by side. It is important to note that neither the soul nor the 'I' have any influence on this process. The life-tableau is simply there to be seen in its fullness.

This stage lasts for approximately three days. Many cultures have a three-day period around death where family and friends tend to the body and pay tribute to the deceased. During this time the vital body gradually dissolves in the etheric mantle surrounding the earth and the panorama becomes weaker until it finally vanishes.

Your vital life body was formed out of the ether surrounding the earth. During this phase, your habits and abilities, such as playing, making music, thinking, etc., dissolve back into the etheric earth field. Physically and vitally, you replace what you borrowed while you lived on the earth.

Emotional body after death: Your emotional/soul body,(sensations, feelings, personality, etc.) and your 'I' spirit now move into the larger planetary world. Here you witness a retrospective view of your life which shows the events you experienced. It is not a tableau, but the actual experiences themselves, starting with your death and moving backwards. Here it is not your own feelings you experience, but rather the feelings you caused others in your social contacts on earth. You experience every joy or pain you have caused others; a complimentary experience of your own deeds. No changes can be made to what has occurred, but a deeper insight into social living is gained.

The impulses and desires which your 'I' could not control during life (i.e. greed for food, addiction to drugs, uncontrollable urges and desires) are now addressed. While the longing is still there, you have no physical body to satisfy it. These unsatisfied desires cause distress. But the soul is not able to loosen itself from the 'I' until those attachments are resolved. This period lasts approximately one-third the length of time of your recent life, corresponding to the amount of time you spent sleeping. Religious traditions refer to this period as purgatory while esoteric traditions refer to it as purification.

Once the soul has resolved its attachments it is ready to loosen itself from its connection to the 'I' and move back into the astral world. However, you do leave behind remnants of unresolved relationships, problems etc. in the astral world.

'I' spirit after death: Now the 'I' is free to widen into the next sphere which is the home of all humankind and your individual core of being. In religious terms it called heaven, or the realm of the Creator, God. Here a meeting takes place with your higher 'I'; the part of your 'I' that never fully incarnated on earth. What remains with you from your most recent earth-life are the capacities that your 'I' achieved during life on earth. These are spiritual virtues such as patience, empathy, focused attention, the ability to love.

The results of living on earth enriched and perfected your higher 'I'—which is the true essence of who you are. You will meet the 'Judge', spiritual powers that created you, who will evaluate and put into order your newly acquired faculties.

In the process some gaps may be noted which will form a blueprint for future development. In this way the impulse for your next incarnation and its tasks come about. A 'draft plan' is made from the vantage point of the spiritual world, but not all details are determined. It points to particular faculties that need to be developed or refined in order to resolve earthly entanglements and fashion new relationships going forward. This completes the life cycle.

A path towards the earth: Time and effort is now spent on working out the plans for shaping a new physical body with characteristics that will be ideal for the lessons to be learned in the next incarnation. With the insights gained in the review process, your 'I' spirit now takes the responsibility of self-development going forward. A new life on earth is needed to allow for experiences that foster the desired development. As a reincarnated human being, we are limited to a physical body, but our 'I' consciousness, which thinks and chooses, remains independent of earthly influences. Thus, your 'I' makes decisions and takes responsibility for them when on earth. Therein lies the human freedom to choose, to err, to learn and correct and to become accountable.

As your 'I' spirit sets out to return to earth, the path leads back through the planetary world. Your soul composition is newly arranged to form the emotional/soul body for your next incarnation. The residue you left behind is incorporated for further work as your 'I' attaches itself more strongly to your soul. Connected, these two bodies draw closer to earth, watching for the chance of physical incarnation which is suitable for what the soul and spirit require. Conception begin a new incarnation; a new life has begun.

The value of understanding reincarnation lies in the fact that human beings, as we appear on earth, are not a matter of chance. Every incarnation is the result of all past lives plus extensive planning and development prior to return. We come with all of our problems and past errors to address (karma), as well as the many gifts and capacities we have.

This rich mix of being human will have many chances to grow and develop further in each successive lifetime.

PREPARING FOR DEATH

What is your attitude towards death? Some fear it, others ignore it, while still others prepare for it. The more consciously we live our life, the more progress can be made in death. The best preparation for death is to clear up the negative energy in your life as much as possible. Prepare for death by dealing with your life.

o *Do a life audit:* A bibliography review is an ideal way to review the various aspects of your life; experiences, relationships, successes and failures, cravings and compulsions, acts of kindness and generosity, contributions and injury to others (See Section II). See it all by being as honest as possible. Also, be as celebratory about your greatness as you are judging about your shortcomings. A balanced approach is most helpful— and honest.

o *Make amends:* Wherever you find unfinished business, make an effort to clear it up. Ask for forgiveness from those you have wronged. Express gratitude to those who have touched your life in an unforgettable manner. Forgive those who have hurt you. Return what you have borrowed. Complete promises made. Wrap up loose ends, whatever and wherever they may be.

o *Become balanced:* Where are your excesses? Identify any cravings or unsatisfied deep desires you still deal with. Recognize what you love and what you hate. See where you are clear or irrational in your beliefs and expectations. Learn how to be open and flexible, connected yet detached. Finding the meaning in an unsettling thought or event is the activity that will create a balanced view. Get into 'right relationship' with all things in your life.

o *Make plans:* The kindest thing we can do for our loved
ones is make plans for our funeral. Make physical
arrangement such as a living will or healthcare power of
attorney. Gather up all legal and financial papers in one
place (will, insurance papers, etc.) as well as contact
information. Also, do relationship planning for the end
of life. Identify who you have messages for and call
them, or write a note to be delivered upon your death.
Select special objects for certain people and deliver them,
or label them so that they can be given to the recipient
upon your death. Plan for your pet when you die.

An Example of Death by Completion

My first patient encounter as a student nurse taught me
about conscious living; it was a career-altering moment for
me. I did not fully appreciate its impact on my life until I had
the privilege of assisting my mother in the final months and
days of her life.

As a nursing student, my first patient taught me about
living—in her dying. Four months into my nursing program
we had worked diligently in the nursing lab, testing our skills
in admissions, injections, bathing. And finally the day came
for our first day of clinical experience. I was assigned to 3
North Medical; the patient in room 312. My role was
straightforward; simply admit her and fill out the necessary
forms. "Simple enough", I thought to myself.

I shyly tapped on the door and entered her room. This
most beautiful woman, age 75, was sitting on the edge of her
bed. I was struck by her serenity and presence. After the
required introduction, I asked "What brought you to the
hospital?" She looked at me with blue piercing eyes, glinting
with a bit of humor, and said, "My children". "Oh! And why
do they think you should be in the hospital?" I inquired
further. "They think I am crazy" she mentioned in an
offhanded way.

Immediately I conjured up images of 'mental illness'.
"And why do they think you are crazy?" I continued.
"Because I told them that I am going to die". Something
about all of this was almost surreal. I truly looked at her, and
there was not a hint of a body ravaged by illness, no agitation
or emotion other than deep peace.

I began again, as my paper was still blank. "So what are
you dying of, if I may ask." "Completion—I am dying of
completion", was her soft reply. In that instant I felt this
deep shift within my body. I was all of 18 years old, new to
this whole field of work, but intuitively I KNEW that I was
witnessing something extra-ordinary.

"I'm sorry, but I am not sure I understand. Could you say
a little more about that?" I prodded. She went on to tell me
about the wonderful life she had lived. She had just made the
rounds to all of her children, spending a week with each one
of them. On that trip she had taken some of their treasures
she had kept for years, as well as a few

meaningful things from her own collection. She told them
each how proud she was of them, how much she loved them.
She had said 'all she had to say.' Then, she went on to
explain, she made a list of all the people that she had to touch
base with to 'wrap things up'. She itemized things; people
she wanted to thank, those she wanted to apologize to, those
she had business dealings or financial matters left to finish.
She went through each aspect of her life, and put it all in
order. So, here was this beautiful, lucid and peaceful woman,
expressing deep gratitude for her wonderful life, and a
readiness to surrender it all in a graceful passing. She had
truly done her personal life work.

I went back to the desk where the Instructor was
waiting—page empty. When she asked what the patient was
being admitted for, I answered, "Death by Completion".
Needless to say she was MOST disappointed, critical of my
interviewing skills and gave me a double reading assignment
in the library in preparation for clinical rotation the following
day.

Returning to my dorm room, I was simply filled with the wonder of that exchange. The next day I was assigned to someone else, but I started my rounds in her room. There she was! Sitting in a chair, she was smiling and serene and very much as she had been the day before. I reviewed her chart—all tests showed normal. The next day I returned again, only to find her room empty. When I inquired at the desk—she had died the night before of 'natural causes'. I would have added—death by completion.

Chapter 10

Creating a Healthy Life Pattern:
Whole health by design

> You must understand the whole of life,
> not just one little part of it. That is why you
> must read, that is why you must look at the
> skies, that is why you must sing and dance,
> and write poems, and suffer and
> understand, for all of that is life.
> Jiddu Krishamurti

What is the first thing you do upon awakening? What is the last thing you do before sleeping? And how do you fill the days of your life? How much of your life is lived in mindlessness and how much of it is consciously focused? Human beings feel and know themselves as individuals only when they awaken to full awareness. With the help of clear thinking and purposeful planning we can design a life that is health-promoting, personally fulfilling and life-enhancing for others as well.

Like the rest of nature, human nature needs to have rhythms and patterns in its life. Rhythm creates vitality. Creating and maintaining a healthy lifestyle will keep you vibrantly healthy and energetic. Engaging with art, music or inspiring thoughts will keep you centered. Establishing moments of quiet each day to empty your mind and quiet your thoughts will keep you grounded. And living from a place of purposeful awareness will keep you free—to live an authentic self-directed life rather than adopting or responding to the rules and whims of the outer world. This is the path to wholeness.

WORKING OUT - STRENGTHENING THE BODY

Remember that your amazing human body has 4 qualities—each with its own intelligence (Physical, Vital Energy, Emotional Soul and , Mind/ "I"). A total fitness program must address them all. Your physical and vital body are inseparable; think of them as an integrated unit.

Mineral Physical Body: Qualities of your physical body include:

- Elements of the earth (air, water, minerals, chemicals)
- Gives form & structure to the body (skeleton, muscles, organs)
- Carries potential for decay and destruction (metabolism, catabolism)
- *Mechanical Intelligence—provides balance & movement*
- Activities to strengthen it: nutrition, exercise, safety & rest

Care of the physical body is a well-known path to fitness; nutrition and exercise programs abound. Find one that fits your lifestyle and your temperament—and enjoy it!

Plant Vitality Body: Qualities of your vital energy body include:

- Supports the 7 Vital Life Processes:(*Taking In:* breathing, warming, nourishing; *Processing:* secreting, regulating, reproducing; growing)
- Complete life cycle: birth, growth, decline, death (cardio-vascular, brain & CNS, GI/GU systems)
- Reproduces its own kind (reproductive & endocrine systems)

145

- *Energetic Intelligence—provides vitality & potentiates life processes*
- Activities to strengthen it: organic foods & herbs, massage, acupuncture, yoga, hot/cold packs, outdoor/garden meditations

Care of the vital body focuses on enhancement of the rhythmic processes that support health and unify the body. A hallmark of all living things, as opposed to a purely mechanical system such as your physical body, is that an activity or change in one area always exerts some influence on every other part of the organism. This principle applies strongly in practices such as acupuncture and reflexology. An interconnection between nervous stimulation in the muscles and emotional disturbances can lead to muscular tension, a loss of fluidity, and a tendency towards rigidity. Massage affects and softens the skin and underlying muscles and soft tissue. Plant oils applied directly or through the use of warm or cold packs, enhance circulation, regulation and secretion at all levels of the body. Heat is often used to stimulate the healing properties of the body, while also providing warmth and enhanced circulation. Stretching programs such as yoga increase flexibility and fluidity.

Energy Anatomy Grid
5 Distinct Layers

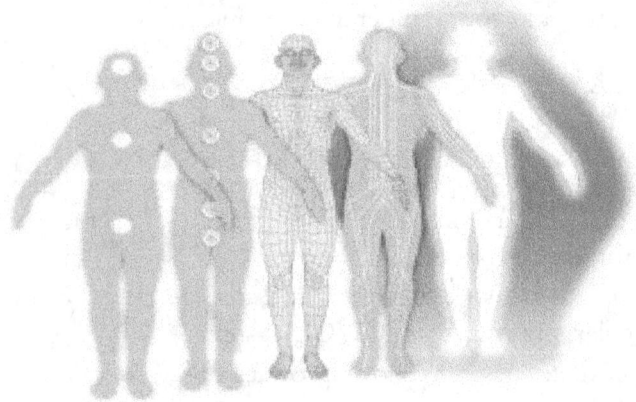

<u>Energy Increasing Practices: Working with Your Energy System:</u>

Your physical/vital body focuses on 'energetic anatomy': interconnected 'energy fields' that provide the vital life force to the human body. It is made up of 5 layers that create an energy grid: http://www.soundstrue.com/shop/The-Power-of-Energy-Healing/3266.pd

- <u>Energy Flow & Balance</u>: You can increase your energy—in real time—by one of the following:
  - o   Tracing or swirling the hand over the body along specific energy pathways – massage or acupuncture
  - o   Using specific exercises or postures such as yoga or stretching
  - o   Surrounding an area with healing energies, aromatherapy, plant oils, heat, compassionate support in stress (one person's energies impact another's)
  - o   Drumming, massaging, twisting, or connecting to specific energy points on the body

Energy Tapping
Chest Exercise

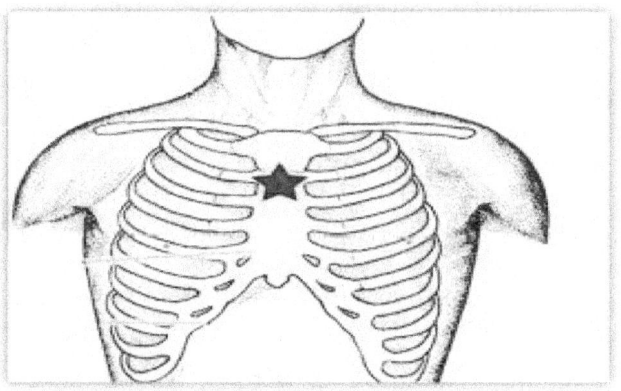

- <u>Tapping Exercise:</u> When feeling tired or sluggish you can 'boost' your energy in the following ways:

- o *Chest Method:* Tap for 2-5 minutes on chest mid-sternum
- o *Front of Body Method:* Tap in succession down extremities & trunk for 2-5 minutes
- o *Back Method:* Tap the back of your colleague for 2-5 minutes and then exchange positions

- Breath Watch: Relax your entire body, and with closed eyes:
  - o Inhale slowly through your nostrils & imagine a pure white cloud filling your lungs—5 counts.
  - o Suspend breathing for 5 counts, watching clean air travel to all extremities. is.
  - o Exhale the smoky de-oxygenated cloud thru your nostrils & see it disappear—5 counts.
  - o Suspend breath for 5 counts, feeling the emptiness in your lungs & feet extending into the earth for grounding.
  - o Repeat 10 more times & notice the calm relaxation take over.

Six Vital Energy Practices:
1. Consume Raw Energy: Be the stove—go natural
2. Connect to Nature: Breathe in fresh air, ground yourself, expose yourself to sunlight
3. Move Your Body: Walk (Whenever you can; on phone, during TV commercial etc.), Stretch out (Stand tall & lengthen your step), Tap (Awaken your energy), Tuck (Buttocks tucked & shoulders broad, bend down as far as is comfortable)
4. Breathe Deeply—to count of 5 (Inhale, Hold, Exhale, Hold)
5. Express and FEEL Gratitude: Practice feeling the wave of energy that flows through you when you practice positive thinking
6. BE a positive energy source for others (share your wisdom & support others efforts)

WORKING THROUGH - STRENGTHENING THE SOUL

Emotional/Soul Body: Qualities of your emotional body include:

- Bridge between outer world (physical/vital bodies) and inner world (conscious mind/spirit)

- Brain and CNS provides movement and action.

- Logical Mind—home of ego and personality, receives sensations and impressions from outer world and forms an emotional feeling which guides a reaction based on instincts, drives, habits or rational choice

- Links to higher mind for conscious choice, or reactionary brain for quick response

- _Emotional Intelligence—combines emotional understanding (of self and other) with intelligence when making a decision_

- Activities to strengthen it: art, music, color, sound, movement, poetry, sculpture

In past societies, painting, music, sculpture and architecture were considered sacred activities. Art forms arrange and adapt images of the physical world in such a way that they have a strong impact on human emotions and the creation of meaning. Artistic modalities connect with the emotional aspect of the soul and the 'meaning making' aspects if the human spirit.

Lovers of music have a sense of the expression of their higher spirit, or find support for sadness or joy in a particular song or sound. Colors and symbols in paintings, like music, evoke expression of powerful feelings, while movement and dance express emotions and rhythms through the physical body. Sculpture work done with clay can be very grounding for an agitated state. The sense of rhythm in speech is expressed in poetry. Enlivening the rhythm in the soul can have a very therapeutic effect. Engaging in the fine arts is a therapeutic way to express and strengthen the emotional body. Art, music, sculpture, pottery, weaving, music, poetry and dance are all modalities to get in touch with, and express, your emotions.

Soul Enhancing Practices: Working with Your Emotional System:

- Emotional Energy Balance: Grasp finger with thumb underneath & 4 fingers wrapped around it, resting on the top of the thumb:

Emotional Energy Balance
Acupressure

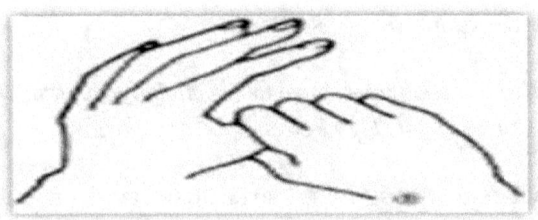

For Emotional Challenge: (Hold each finger for 1 minute)

- o Thumb: Worry
- o Second Finger: Fear
- o Middle Finger: Anger
- o Forth Finger: Grief
- o Fifth Finger: Pretense

For Stress/Fear: (Hold for 3 minutes)
- o Press Thumb into palm of hand
- o Press 4 fingers into back of the hand
- o Take three deep breaths

- Engaging in the Fine Arts:
  - o *Creative Arts* – take a class or pursue a hobby in painting, sculpture, weaving, pottery, book study,

handicrafts, woodworking, gardening, photography, bird watching, camping in nature

o   *Expressive Arts*- Learn a dance step, how to play piano or a musical instrument, write poetry, prose or stories, journal

o   *Art Appreciation* – develop a playlist of various music categories to support your various moods, get a seasons ticket to the theater, attend movies and concerts, take classes on the history of jazz or Broadway, study the life of famous authors or artists

Six Soul Enhancing Practices:
When an emotion arises, catch yourself before you react, take a deep breath and let reason replace habit—practice emotional intelligence

1.   Listen to music, matching the type of songs to the activities or mood of the moment and practice noticing how the rhythms and sounds 'flow' in waves into your body
2.   Learn the energy points on your hand that reduce stress, fear or anger, and use them when in a meeting or with others in a potentially stressful situation
3.   Take up a hobby that allows you to be creative and expressive; dance, sing, write, sculpt
4.   Fine tune your senses so that you can pick up on things in your environment before they become too developed and hard to reverse; develop mindfulness
5.   Practice Emotional Intelligence in your relationships
6.   Practice the art of tolerance and appreciation—it is the best antidote to emotional challenges

WORKING IN – STRENGTEHING THE SPIRIT

While the other three human capacities are connected to the physical body, the spirit is in another realm. Your mind is a two-fold entity: Lower Mind which lives in your soul and engages the outer world; and Higher Mind which lives in your spirit and engages in your inner world. 'I' is the consistent witness and director of the activities between these two worlds and the two conscious/thinking (choosing and acting) aspects of your Self.

Human Mind/ "I" Spirit:: Qualities of your "I" spirit include:

- Unique to the human species—our conscious self-aware being, unchanging throughout our life, and even death.

- Higher Mind—home of authentic self, spontaneously uses reflection and wisdom, imagination, creativity, intuition, moral and spiritual values that transcend instincts and reactions in choosing a response.

- "I"—our unique and autonomous spirit—our guide who resides in our Inner World which holds all knowledge accumulated throughout this, and other lives

- Fosters intentionally selected, courageous and creative choices throughout life which develops a unique biography, and greater good for society.

- _Spiritual Wisdom—combines logic and intuition with higher knowing, creating truth and beauty_

- Activities to strengthen it: life review based on biographical phases, psychological & spiritual activities, prayer and meditation

As the external world impacts the physical body, the 'I' can clearly and consciously perceive the stirrings of the soul forces and modify them by reflecting on them. Mindfulness, meditation and periods of silence strengthen awareness which fosters our ability to think in a wakeful consciousness. This is enhanced when we are engaged in experiences of the world, sharing thoughts in dialogue with other human beings. It is also necessary to be self-reflective; to think, choose, decide evaluate and carry out responsibility that tests our will, wisdom and capacity for love.

Our 'I' is the personal guide that holds the direction of our life. From outer experiences and inner impressions we create our personal biography and our own history. Thoughtful life review, psychological or spiritual counseling, and other reflective practices strengthen and enhance the insight of our 'I'. This wisdom is passed back to us when we seek silence to hear our inner voice. Pondering the knowledge gained, we can create a focused and relevant response to the challenges and opportunities that come our way.

Spirit Enhancing Practices: Working with Your Mind's 'I':

Several categories should be considered when designing 'spiritual activities' for your health plan: activities that strengthen the connection between your inner and outer world, and a review of your life biography that gives pattern recognition and understanding as a foundation for moving towards your future.

- Outer/Inner World Development Practices: Vital to spiritual growth is strengthening the bridge between experience and understanding through:
  o Games/Reading/Lifelong Learning etc.
  o Perspective-broadening Art: Study it's focus, repetition, perspective, multidimensionality
  o Mind Management: Visualization, Guided Imagery, Meditation, Breath Work, Prayer & Distance Healing, Practice Enhanced Awareness
  o Reduce Ambivalence: confusion drains energy and increases error. Become clear about your goals and intentions and let them guide you in the choices you make

- <u>Biographical Stages of Development:</u> Refer back to Section II for activities and exercises designed to assist with biographical review.

- <u>Reflective Exercise: Reassessing My Life - Why Am I Here?</u>
  At mid-life and beyond the energy shifts from fueling the physical & vital bodies to supporting the development of the emotional and spiritual bodies. IF we are willing to engage the crucial developmental tasks of this shifting time, the second half of life has all the excitement, opportunity and satisfaction our earlier life offered—and more. It can be the most satisfying & gratifying stage of life.
  o What is the purpose of my life; what have I been called to do or contribute?

  o What impact does my life have on current & future generations; for the greater good of all?

  o What parts of my family heritage, traditions or memories do I want to keep alive?

  o What of my heritage must be changed for the positive evolution of the human family?

  o Do I have more or less enthusiasm & motivation for living; regrets or disappointments that weigh me down?

  o To what degree have I developed self-compassion & self-acceptance?

  o What do I want to be remembered <u>as</u>: kind, caring, peaceful etc.?

A key to the practice of wisdom: When things get difficult, replace a response of fear or anger with one of your major intentions; i.e. peace, surrender, gratitude, trust, love, forgiveness etc. Eventually it becomes your response to every life even when things are hard.

- Morning Mind/Spirit Training—Preparing for the Day: Every day is a new beginning. Your task each morning is to learn the practice of entering your body and your day consciously.

o Begin by focusing attention on your entire day, from morning to evening. Review your plans for the day. Think about where you need to be and who you will be with.

o Sense your comfort level. Do you feel stressed about this day or do you feel comfortable? Do you feel prepared for the day's events? Most importantly, are you projecting any fears and/or expectations onto the day?

Wisdom Tip: Remind yourself that we lose power with fears & expectations. We gain power when we come to the situation with an open and creative mind rather than a scripted and conditioned response.

- Evening Mind/Spirit Training—Preparing for the Night: As you prepare for sleep, reflect on the activities of your day.

o Review your day backwards, starting with the present moment

o See yourself from *others point of view*, not your own

o Recall the *outcomes* of your choices/decisions/actions

o Look for patterns in your thoughts, feelings &/or reactions

o Celebrate your efforts and put the day to rest

Wisdom Tip: Remember that reflection creates insight and growth—WISDOM. Ignoring to process and integrate the events in your life sets you up to repeat the same old patterns. Life is then a habit instead of a journey of discovery.

11- <u>Tying Up Loose Ends—Preparation for Completion:</u>
An important practice as we age is healing any negative energy that we are carrying. While some of it is physical in nature, much of it has to do with decisions and relationships that 'missed the mark'. Three simple exercises can help us move through those negative elements in our life:

o   Be mindful of ambivalence: Do not stay undecided. It leads to error and regret. Rather than trying to figure out if 'it' is good or bad (which is what keeps us stuck) cultivate the attitude 'It is what it is'. Once it can be accepted at face value, we will be more clearly focused on the essence of the issue, a response that is appropriate for us to get to the desired outcome. Get rid of ambivalence.

o   Manage betrayal, disappointment & regret: We are human beings programmed to learn by trial and error. Society has evolved into a perfectionistic and blaming culture which makes sincere experimentation difficult for fear of a mistake. Know that you have made many and will continue to make more of them. Identify the people who have hurt you, as well as those you have injured. Make a second list of those who have blessed you. Make connections (face-to-face, phone, letters, e-mail) and express your forgiveness, apology or gratitude. It will lighten your load—and heal a wound on both sides.

o   Replace self-esteem with self-compassion: (Refer back to Chapter 3.) When we develop compassion for ourselves, tolerance and understanding for others follows. We can put away the drive for competition and winner, replacing it instead with the knowing that 'everything is simply a lesson'. Harsh judgment gives way to openness and tolerance. Life becomes a learning and exchanging feast of ideas and experiences. Our biography deepens and our destiny is enriched.

Six Spirit Enhancing Exercises:

During the transition moments of the day and evening one is most open spiritually. It is at these moments we have a clarity that is not as available to us during the rest of the day. When we make it a practice to start and end our day in a conscious way, we learn our greatest lessons and insights from our life experiences.

1. Reexamine your life purpose

2. Reduce ambivalence

3. Practice reverse order recall

4. Reduce judgment, rise above your dis-likes

5. Bring completion to the 'loose ends of your life'

6. Practice your 'intentions' when things get difficult—with gratitude

Putting it All Together:

Create Your Healthy Living Plan to address all four aspects of your 'Self' by completing the following steps:

1. Consider the following as foundational to your plan:
- Life goals; intentions for your 'whole person'
- Motivation for health; i.e. mindfulness program 'lite' or 'heavy'
- Your age; i.e. youth, middle age, older
- Your over-all 'health' and 'fitness'; i.e. BMI, chronicity, stamina
- Your life stage; i.e. student/married/single/working
- Other life responsibilities; i.e. aging parents, young children

- <u>Financial capacity</u>; i.e. healthy foods, gym membership
- <u>Access to resources</u>; i.e. 'exercise' programs, grocery stores
- <u>Commitment level</u>; i.e. how much time/length of plan

2. Select a few activities from each category for over-all fitness. Or, you may choose to focus deeply on one area only that is especially important at this time.

3. Time for your plan: Take a calendar and write your plan into the time and activities going on in your daily life. If it does not fit into an already over-crowded life, chances for success are minimal.

4. Set measurable goals and evaluate yourself periodically—monthly, quarterly etc.

5. Recruit a friend or family member—commitment stays stronger when there is someone else involved.

6. Enjoy a healthy, vibrant and balanced life—YOURS

When we cease to be perfect and accept that we cannot control our lives, we find peace, serenity and joy in our authentic selves. The less defensive we are the more love we experience. It is the moment of true surrender; a beginning of trust in the Universe.

RECOMMENDED READING

Bamford, Christopher, *Start Now! A Book of Soul and Spiritual Exercises*, Massachusetts, Steiner   Books, 2004.

Benner, Patricia, *From Novice to Expert: Excellence and Power in Clinical Nursing Practice,* Prentice Hall, New Jersey 2001.

Bott, Victor, *An Introduction to Anthroposophical Medicine*, Rudolf Steiner Press, Forrest Row 2004.

Bryant, William, *The Veiled Pulse of Time: an Introduction to Biographical Cycles and Destiny, Lindisfarne* Press, New York 1996.

Burkhard, Gudrun, *Biographical Work: the Anthroposophical Basis*, Floris Books, Edinburgh 2007.

___, *Taking Charge: Your Life Patterns and Their Meaning,* Floris Books, Edinburgh, 1997.

Camps, A., Hagenhoff, B., van der Star, A., *Anthroposophical Care for the Elderly,* Floris Books, Edinburgh, 2008.

Childs, Gilbert, *Understanding your Temperament: A Guide to the Four Temperaments,* Sophia Books, London, 2009.

Choquette, Sonia, *The Intuitive Spark,* Hay House, New York, 2007.

Evans, Michael and Ian Rodgers, *Complete Healing,* Steinerbooks, Massachusetts 2005.

Glas, Norbert, *The fulfillment of Old Age*, Anthroposophic Press, New York 1986.

Goldberg, Elkhonon, *The Wisdom Paradox*, Gotham Books, New York, 2006.

Held, Wolfgang, *Rhythms of the Week and Other Explorations of Time*, Floris Books, Edinburgh, 2011.

Houten, Coenraad van, *Awakening the Will: Principles and Processes in Adult Learning,* Temple Lodge Press, Forest Row 2003.

Johnson, Robert, *Inner Work,* Harper Collins, New York, 1986.

Kamm, Laura, *Intuitive Wellness: Using Your Body's Inner Wisdom to Heal,* Atria Books, New York, 2007.

Koerner, JoEllen, *Death by Completion: a Guide to Conscious,* mylifemycanvas, South Dakota 2012.

___, *Healing Presence: the Essence of Nursing,* Springer Publishing, New York, 2011

___, *Mother Heal MySelf: an Intergenerational Healing Journey Between Two Worlds,* Crestport Press, California, 2003.

Kubler-Ross, Elizabeth, *On Death and Dying,* Routledge, London 2008.

Lievegoed, Bernard, *Phases: the Spiritual Rhythms of Adult Life,* Sophia Books, Forrest Row 1998.

___, *Phases of Childhood,* Floris Books, Edinburgh: Anhroposophic Press, New York, 1997.

___, *Man on the Threshold: Challenge of Inner Development,* Hawthorn Press, Stroud 1985.

Levinson, Daniel J., *The Seasons of a Man's Life,* New York, 1979.

Madaus, J.R., *Think Logically, live Intuitively: Seeking the Balance,* Hampton Roads,Virginia,2005.

Margolis, Char, *Disvoer Your Inner Wisdom,* Fireside, New York, 2008.

Moody, Raymond, *Life after Life,* Rider & Co, London, 2001.

Tessa Therkleson, *Nursing the Human Being: An Anthroposophic Perspective,* Mercury Press, New York, 2007.

Sheehy, Gail, *Pathfinders*, New York, 1981.

Soesman, Albert, *Our Twelve Senses: Wellspring of the Soul*, Hawthorn Press, Stroud, 2006.

Steiner, Rudolf, *Anthroposophy and the Inner Life,* London, Rudolf Steiner Press, 1994.

___, *Anthroposophy in Everyday Life*, Anthroposophic Press, Massachusetts, 1995.

___, *Aspects of Human Evolution*, Anthroposophic Press, New York, 1987.

___, *Biography, Freedom and Destiny: Enlightening the Path of Human Life*, Rudolf Steiner Press, London, 2009.

___, *First Steps in Inner Development*, Massachusetts, Anthroposophic Press, 1999.

___,*Getting Old*, Mercury Press, New York, 2009.

___, *How Can Mankind find Christ Again?* Anthroposophic Press, New York 1984

___, *How to Know Higher Worlds: A Modern Path of Initiation*, Anthroposophic Press, New York, 1994.

___, *The Manifestation of Karma*, Rudolf Steiner Press, London 1995.

___, *Inner Reading and Inner Hearing*, Steinerbooks, Massachusetts 2008.

___, *The Meaning of Life*, Rudolf Steiner Press, Forest Row 2005.

___, *An Outline of Esoteric Science,* Anthroposophic Press, New York, 1997.

___, *Philosophy of Freedom*, Rudolf Steiner Press, London 1988.

___, *Reincarnation and Karma*, Anthroposophic Press, New York 1992.

___, *Sleep and Dreams: A Bridge to the Spirit,*

___, *Theosophy*, Anthroposophic Press, New York, 1994.

___, *A Way of Self Knowledge*, Massachusetts Anthroposophic Press 1998.

___, *A Western Approach to Reincarnation and Karma*, Anthroposophic Press, New Your 1997.

Steiner, Rudolf, &Scala, Patsy, *Weekly Meditations: Rodolf Steineir's Calendar of the Soul*, Steiner Books, Forrest Row, 2008.

ABOUT THE AUTHOR

JoEllen Koerner is a nurse entrepreneur and founder of My Life My Canvas, a web-based organization with a special emphasis on holistic health and life balance. Her programs offer tools and strategies that empower people to manage their own health by blending all-inclusive principles of various traditions; indigenous, western, eastern and anthroposophic. Her international and voluntary work is focused on web-enhanced school-community partnerships that support health and life quality for underrepresented sectors of society. Dr. Koerner has published two others books: *Mother Heal MySelf: An intergenerational Healing Journey Between Two Worlds; and Healing Presence: The Essence of Nursing*. She can be reached at- jkoerner@mylifemycanvas.com.